THE · BUSINESS · SIDE · OF · GEPITAL

Making Sense of

F

2 8

0 6

B

a

te

Fi

E
a
t
F
E

© 1991 Radcliffe Medical Press Ltd
15 Kings Meadow, Ferry Hinksey Road, Oxford OX2 0DP

Reprinted 1991

British Library Cataloguing in Publication Data
Making sense of audit.
   1. Great Britain. General Practice. Auditing
   I. Irvine, Donald   II. Irvine, Sally   III. Series
   657.834

   ISBN 1 870905 12 1

Typeset by Acorn Bookwork, Salisbury
Printed and bound in Great Britain by
Biddles Ltd, Guildford and King's Lynn

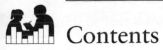

Contents

Foreword

The term audit was first introduced into medicine as recently as forty years ago although the idea that medical practitioners would analyse the work they did and assess the benefits is much older. The first systematic analyses were introduced — in 1912 — not by physicians but by surgeons in the USA.

However, the concept is even older than that. Hippocrates, sitting under the great tree of his on the island of Cos, reported on the outcome of the diseases of all the patients he saw. But then philosophy took over from science in medicine and little further progress was made for nearly 2000 years.

Nevertheless, there were some who expressed the hope the doctors should be more analytical about their activities, but progress was slow. Francis Bacon, in the 16th century, wrote on the subject, and a century and a half later, Francis Clifton made a plea for hospital medical records to be published so that the data therein could be analysed. He even listed the headings under which the analyses could be carried out:

1. Sexus, aetas, species, temeries, occupatio, et victus aegri
2. Dies morbi
3. Morbi phenomena
4. Dies mensis
5. Remedia
6. Effectus

which, in translation, means:

1. Sex, age, type, temperament, occupation and diet
2. Duration of disease
3. The symptoms of the disease
4. The day of the month
5. Remedy (treatment)
6. Effect (of the treatment)

Clifton went on to say: 'The benefit the public would receive (from such disclosures) would vastly more than balance the expense.'

A hundred years later in the early 19th century Wakely founded the Lancet and, in it, he wrote numerous trenchant editorials. In one, written in 1841 he said: 'All public institutions should be compelled to keep casebooks and registers. ... Annual abstracts of results must be published (and these must embrace hospitals, lying-in dispensaries, lunatic asylums and prisons'. Dispensaries were the precursors of health centres; so, clearly, had Wakely been writing today, he would have extended medical audit to include general practice.

Audit is now an accepted part of medical care; indeed it is an integral feature of the new NHS, both in general and hospital practice. With audit goes quality assurance; the right of the consumer (ie the patient) and the purchaser (which, in the NHS is the Government) to expect a reasonable standard from the providers of service.

The editors of this book are both experienced practitioners, Sally Irvine in the field of management and Donald Irvine in general practice. The result is a very readable guide to audit.

STUART CARNE

List of Contributors

JAMES COX, FRCGP, MICGP, *General Practitioner, Caldbeck, Cumbria; Associate Adviser in General Practice, University of Newcastle upon Tyne*

PAUL CREIGHTON, FRCGP, *General Practitioner, The Health Centre, Broomhill, Northumberland; Associate Adviser in General Practice, University of Newcastle upon Tyne*

LYNN GRAHAM, LL B, ACA, *Practice Manager, Guidepost Medical Group, Northumberland*

ALLEN HUTCHINSON, FRCGP, *Director, Ambulatory Care Programme, Centre for Health Services Research, University of Newcastle upon Tyne*

DONALD IRVINE, CBE, MD, FRCGP, *General Practitioner, Lintonville Medical Group, Ashington, Northumberland; Regional Adviser in General Practice, University of Newcastle upon Tyne*

SALLY IRVINE, MA (Cantab), *General Administrator, Royal College of General Practitioners, London; President, Association of Health Centre and Practice Administrators*

COLIN LEON, MBE, FRCGP, *formerly General Practitioner, Gateshead, Tyne and Wear; formerly Associate Adviser in General Practice, University of Newcastle upon Tyne*

GEORGE TAYLOR, FRCGP, MICGP, DRCOG, *General Practitioner, Guidepost Medical Group, Northumberland; Associate Adviser in General Practice, University of Newcastle upon Tyne*

ROGER THORNHAM, FRCGP, *General Practitioner, Norton Medical Centre, Stockton-on-Tees; Associate Adviser in General Practice, University of Newcastle upon Tyne*

The Business Side of General Practice

Editorial Board

Acknowledgements

WE are extremely grateful to the practices of all the contributors for allowing their colleagues to draw freely on their experiences of audit.

The staff of the Division for General Practice within the Regional Postgraduate Institute for Medicine and Dentistry in the University of Newcastle upon Tyne have been helpful and supportive throughout, and we thank them.

Above all, we are deeply indebted to Mrs Jill Mitchell who has cheerfully accomplished an immense amount of typing in a very short space of time.

DONALD AND SALLY IRVINE
May 1991

Section I

1 Introduction

AUDIT is the process used by health professionals to assess, evaluate and improve the care of patients in a systematic way in order to enhance their health and quality of life.

This book begins with a description of audit, giving an account of its benefits and uses, and of the methods available to carry it out. The basic data requirements of different types of audit are discussed, as is the analysis of results, and how to bring about change in the practice.

The reader could stop there. However the second part of the book (Section II) continues with a collection of case histories from the contributors' general practices. Each history summarizes a working audit of a particular practice which was carried out to help overcome practical problems and to secure improvements. All of the case histories are simple, but they show what can be done with a little thought and imagination, the expenditure of a modest amount of effort and money, and without the need for extensive technical knowledge and skill or the employment of external professionals. Those who feel daunted by the mystique of audit may take encouragement from them!

These case histories, together with the examples cited in the opening chapters, show how general practices attempting to provide a well-defined range of services use audit as a tool which is as indispensable to the delivery of patient care as a stethoscope or the medical records system. Audit also has the potential to be one of the most important factors for improving the health of the community. Moreover, audit can result in patients being more content with the services they receive, and it can encourage conscientious doctors, nurses and receptionists to improve their professional skills, thereby contributing to the smooth running of a practice.

Audit and practice management

The book also sets out to demonstrate that, in three fundamental respects, there is an explicit and direct connection between audit and the way a practice is managed:

1 in the definition of objectives and setting of standards;
2 in the monitoring and assessment of performance;
3 in the management of change.

Modern general practices are now beginning to use the development or business plan as an important mechanism for determining their future direction. From this they can derive their objectives, the main activities necessary to achieve them, and the criteria and standards that indicate good care. The process of defining clinical and operational objectives, criteria and standards is not only the starting point of the management cycle; it is also the starting point of the audit cycle.

The methods and techniques involved in carrying out simple audits within the setting of the individual practice are based on the same principles as those used in practice management for routine performance monitoring. They both require the collection and analysis of practice data, and the comparison of the results against what are understood to be or have been explicitly stated as the practice objectives for care.

Audit may indicate the need for change; management is the process within a practice whereby change is achieved. Moreover audit may also be a powerful and effective tool for bringing about change in an acceptable and workable manner, because it provides reliable up-to-date facts about a practice and its performance, the starting point for effective decision-making. This is especially so when the need for change may not be obvious to or accepted by all members of the practice, or where it is going to involve demanding or uncomfortable adjustments by some individuals.

Audit and management are complementary, largely overlapping, functions. Together they constitute the foundation upon which a practice team can assure quality. Using audit to assure quality helps a practice team to understand the extent to which one team member is dependent upon the quality of work of the others, and also the degree of accountability that all members of the team have to the people who are registered with their practice. Self-sufficiency, self-reliance and self-discipline are attributes associated with quality care and quality management. The case studies reveal how these attributes appeal to health professionals who are keen to exercise considerable freedom of responsibility in the care of patients, without excessive direction from outside. Pragmatically, practice teams who have a positive approach to quality are more likely to secure the funding for their services in future.

The aim throughout this book has been to present audit in as straight-forward and logical way as possible. Purists may feel that the subject has been oversimplified, but the presentation of audit in all its complexity may dampen the enthusiasm of all but the most persistent. Those who are less experienced at audit may be stimulated to explore the subject further as a result of savouring early personal success in the use of audit in their own practices.

2 The Benefits of Audit, or Why Do It

ATTITUDES to audit tend to be coloured by the possible ways in which people think it may be used. For example, when audit is presented as an educational tool, designed to help doctors identify more clearly where they may need new knowledge and skills, or where they could improve their practice, it is generally seen by the medical profession in a positive and encouraging light — a 'good thing'. On the other hand, when audit is perceived as an instrument of health service management, perhaps to check on work done or to cut costs, it is more likely to be regarded as threatening because the results may lead to unacceptable and imposed change.

The trouble with both these common perceptions is that they may result in audit being marginalized by the members of the practice because it is not seen as directly relevant to the mainstream of their daily work in general practice. Either way audit could end up as a fringe activity, to be handled separately from, rather than as an integral part of, normal practice life.

For any practice team contemplating audit the obvious starting point to stimulate interest and activity is therefore to look at the possible benefits for team members and their patients. Positive commitment is critical to motivation. Practice teams who can see audit as a process that is likely to help them, because they recognise its relevance to their work, are likely to invest the time, thought and effort necessary to make it succeed. However, practice teams who see no such benefits are likely to consider audit, at best, as another administrative imposition and intrusion on their lives.

The benefits of audit to a practice are listed in Box 2.1. They are those which the contributors have identified as the most important in improving care for their patients and in enhancing the quality of their professional lives.

The list is by no means exhaustive; nor is it set out in any particular order; nor are the divisions between the benefits discrete. In real life, the benefits of any audit usually cover more than one of the areas listed. Indeed, members of a practice will want to construct their own lists of desired benefits and the act of agreeing on a list will help practice teams to consolidate their reasons for investing in audit.

Reducing frustration

The immediate and most obvious benefit of audit, particularly for health professionals, is the chance it offers to alleviate or remove those areas of

---

Box 2.1: The benefits of audit to a practice

- Reducing frustration
- Bringing about change
- Reducing organizational and clinical error
- Improving efficiency
- Improving effectiveness
- Demonstrating good care
- Meeting patients' needs and expectations
- Stimulating education
- Promoting higher standards of hospital and community care for patients
- Bidding for resources
- Securing effective medical defence through risk avoidance

---

everyday practice that cause frustration. For a practice in which some partners are sceptical about the value of audit, this benefit can be a persuasive motivator. Every practice has problems that everyone complains about but no-one can solve. By defining, quantifying and analysing a problem during audit, solutions may emerge which can then be assessed for their effectiveness through a second audit.

Three simple, yet familiar, situations are presented in Examples 2.1–2.3.

Example 2.1

In every practice, there are occasions when notes required for a consultation are missing.

An audit would reveal why this is happening and point to ways of improving the situation.

Example 2.2

There are always patients who do not attend surgery yet fail to cancel their appointments, which is especially frustrating when other people are waiting for appointments.

An audit would indicate:

- who these non-attenders are;
- whether there are any common patterns;
- how these patients might be persuaded to change;
- whether the persuading techniques introduced actually work.

Example 2.3

Every practice has its 'heart-sink' patients.
  An audit would show:

- who they are;
- how many there are;
- whether they have any common characteristics;
- whether there may be better ways of managing them.

A further example is given in Case Study 10, which shows how a practice used the appointment of a new practice manager to find out what was causing frustration and irritation within the practice team.

Bringing about change

A commonly held belief is that general practitioners are conservative by nature. Young partners often find this to be the case and may turn to colleagues outside the practice for support (one of the main reasons for the interest in young practitioner groups around the country). Historically, the impetus for significant change in most general practices has come from external pressures and circumstances. The New Contract is an obvious example as are the changes needed to become a training practice.

Much time and energy may be expended in partnerships and practice teams in discussing the need for change with little idea of how to bring it about, especially if change is sought by only one or two partners, or the practice manager. The difficulty is compounded if the discussion is based on individual opinion — often passionately held — rather than hard data. In these situations, accurate written descriptions of the current position, and data derived from a practice audit, should give all concerned a clear picture of what is happening. Indeed this is often the key to the way forward.

Example 2.4

The partners of a busy practice in a deprived area felt demoralized by their inability to handle the working day more effectively. Time for patients was too frequently foreshortened, patients too often complained of long waiting times for appointments, and receptionists tended to be caught between pressed doctors and irritated patients. At various times, the cause of the problem was said to be:

- a higher than average patient demand;
- the impact of outside appointments on doctor availability in the practice;
- the organization of the working day around a traditional pattern of two surgeries per partner;
- too little time (6 minutes) for the patient in the consulting room;
- a higher than average list size;
- an unspoken feeling that some partners worked harder than others;
- an uncritical attitude to delegation.

All these factors, singly or in combination, may have been contributory causes. Eventually, and in exasperation the decision was made to collect comprehensive data on doctor availability, the pattern of surgeries, patient demand, workload and the time needed for outside work and non-clinical activities within the practice. From this audit, a complete picture was obtained.

It became clear that the real reason for the partners' inability to manage the working day effectively was due to the lack of unambiguous statements that explicitly defined minimum standards for patient access, and for the length of the average consultation consistent with good care. Defining such standards had to be the starting point, and the following minimum standards were adopted for patients attending the surgery.

- Patients needing emergency treatment will be seen immediately.
- Patients needing an urgent appointment will be seen as soon as possible on the same day.
- Patients requiring a non-urgent appointment with any doctor will be seen within 48 hours.
- The time allocated for the routine consultation will be 10 minutes.

In the event, the following changes were made and solved the problem:

- the 10-minute consultation was implemented;
- the two-surgery day was abandoned in favour of continuous consulting with appropriate breaks;
- more work was delegated to practice nurses;
- further doctor time was made available;
- activities outside the practice were put on a common self-funding basis.

This example illustrates that fitful attempts at symptomatic relief do not solve the problem any more than the symptomatic treatment of disease effects a cure. What does help is an audit to count and classify actual activities in some detail, thus building up a complete picture from which a diagnosis can be made and options for solving the problems can be identified. Case Studies 8 and 9 are further examples of this very common practice situation which can be helped by audit.

Reducing organizational and clinical error

Conscientious health professionals are interested in trying to reduce or eliminate the chances of obvious error. Such concern may save lives and prevent unnecessary stress or suffering; it may also protect the doctor or nurse from litigation, if things go bady wrong. Errors can occur either as a result of a single failure, such as a missed diagnosis, or the wrong choice of treatment, or repeatedly, because of a flaw in a practice system or through ignorance or a persistent deficiency.

· The distinction between organizational and clinical error is largely artificial because both have a direct impact on patient management. In Case Study 11 a confidential enquiry method of audit was used to reduce both types of error.

Efforts to reduce error may bring a practice team closer together by promoting a better understanding within the team. Discussion of the results will raise further questions, some of which may require clarification by repeating the audit in a more specific way.

In the future, the challenge of minimizing error in a practice will become every member's remit as practice teams assume collective responsibility for quality and standards.

Organizational error

Most practices have a shrewd idea of where there may be errors in their organization (*see* Box 2.2).

Box 2.2: Potential organizational errors

- Practice recall systems may be faulty, and so patients may slip through, especially if they have defaulted on an earlier appointment.
- Inconsistencies in the process of handling cervical cytology reports can lead to positive smears being overlooked.
- Patients on long-term drug therapy using repeat prescriptions can be lost to follow-up if there is no effective system for triggering review.
- The doctor may miss 'return' visits to patients if there is no adequate system for follow-up.

A more detailed example is given in Case Study 8, in which the appointment of a deputy practice manager did not achieve the desired objectives. A review showed how a faulty management process led to an incorrect decision and thereby an inappropriate change.

Clinical error

The principle of reducing clinical error is similar to that of reducing organizational error.

Audit can reveal the extent to which a practice meets its criteria and standards for patient care, and thereby reduces the chances of clinical error (*see* Box 2.3).

Box 2.3: Potential clinical errors

- Audits of drug compliance, especially the extent to which therapeutic serum levels are achieved, for example, in the treatment of thyroid deficiency and epilepsy.
- Audits of clinical management, such as determining the action taken on abnormal HbA_1 levels in diabetic patients or significant elevation of the blood pressure in hypertensive patients.
- The avoidance of inappropriate delay in the diagnosis of life-threatening or potentially disabling disease.

Such audits also provide the least painful method of helping colleagues who have a problem (usually a lack of knowledge/skill or an attitude that leads to inappropriate behaviour) to identify, and see what they need to do to put it right.

Improving efficiency

Efficiency is important to any practice, but especially a busy one. Practices by their very nature handle large numbers of people daily, and are substantially demand-led. To make the most efficient use of resources, audits have an important function in practice management and can yield measurable improvements (*see* Examples 2.5–2.7). In Case Study 1, audit was used to improve the efficiency of an 'over-75' screening programme, and in Case Study 14 it was employed to assess the efficiency of a rubella immunization programme.

Example 2.5

An audit of routine data on patterns of doctor-initiated surgery attendances revealed a significant variation among partners in the rates of
'return' consultations. This variation could not be accounted for by
differences in the demographic characteristics of patients attending or the
nature of the illnesses. A further audit pinpointed the main cause, which
was differences in the basis on which each doctor decided whether and
when the patient should return.

Using this information, the partners reviewed their decision-making
process and formulated guidelines to ensure more consistency in future.
Subsequent monitoring (or audit) showed that one partner had increased
the return rate, two had not altered their rate and three had reduced
them. The new basis for bringing patients back was thought to be more
appropriate — at least it could be better justified — and the overall return
rate was reduced, reflecting an improvement in efficiency.

Example 2.6

A practice manager, noting the time it took for some partners to send off
their insurance 'short-reports', initiated a simple, prospective audit
designed to show the time lapse between receipt of the request and
dispatch of the report, partner by partner.

The partners were surprised at how long the delays were, and therefore
became aware of the potential loss of income to the practice. An explicit
protocol to ensure prompt return was introduced, and the practice
manager was asked to continue periodic audits, to monitor individual
compliance.

Example 2.7

A practice was concerned at the number of times patients returned for
appointments to discuss X-ray reports, the results of which were not
available. The practice carried out a short, prospective audit to find out
why.

The result, including associated enquiries, showed that the cause of the
delay lay partly in the length of time it took for the reports to be typed in
the hospital typing pool, and partly in the inefficient filing system in the
practice office which meant that, although the results had been received,
they may not have been filed in the right place. As a consequence, an

explicit standard was defined for the practice, but it was difficult for the practice to have significant influence on the hospital typing system.

Subsequent periodic checks showed that the changes made in the practice office were successful. No changes were noted in the hospital typing pool. However, recent changes in the NHS have meant that the hospital has had to define an explicit standard for reporting its results, and thereby improve its turn-round time.

Future audits carried out by the practice will show whether there has been any further improvement.

Improving effectiveness

In the long term, effectiveness is more relevant to improved patient care than efficiency. Effectiveness equates with outcome; it demonstrates the extent to which a practice's objectives for improving patients' health care are met. Case Studies 1, 5 and 12 are good examples of this.

Example 2.8

A busy urban practice, which had many deprived children registered with it, accepted the need for effective immunization in childhood. The immunization rate was seen by the partners as an appropriate measure of success since a high degree of acquired immunity would eliminate the infections against which protection was being given.

Despite this acceptance, periodic audits over several years showed less than optimum immunization rates. Lack of improvement was largely attributed to the difficulty of gaining access to some of the deprived children. However, it became obvious that this was being used as an excuse; the practice's tracking systems were found to be inadequate and the working practices inflexible. Furthermore, no single person had been assigned responsibility for implementing an immunization programme and therefore no-one was accountable.

The New Contract provided a stimulus to assign responsibility for the programme, to sort out the system and to find new ways of ensuring that children who had defaulted previously were immunized. Further audits showed a progressive improvement such that the practice was able to meet the higher contract targets comfortably.

Periodic audits have now been abandoned in favour of continuous performance monitoring so that the practice knows exactly where it stands on a day to day basis. The current immunization rate for children under 2 years of age is 94%.

The situation in Example 2.8 illustrates three points.

1 The futility of doing audits when no appropriate action is taken, even when the practice team was clear about the direction in which it wanted to go.
2 The impact of an external stimulus (in this case the New Contract) to resolve a problem that had already been identified.
3 The decision by the practice team to abandon periodic audit in favour of continuous monitoring; although the data collected are the same, they have become part of the management cycle to ensure that the practice maintains immunization at the level of optimum effectiveness.

Efficiency studies are easier to mount than effectiveness studies because indicators of efficiency are easier to select and measure than those of effectiveness. However, practice teams need to assess both if their aims are for high standards and the lowest appropriate costs. Case Study 14 is an example of an audit that dealt with both.

Demonstrating good care

Demonstrating good care is one of the traditional uses of audit. However, there is some controversy over whether it makes the best use of a practice's time and resources.

Those who favour demonstrating good care argue that it is insufficient for a practice team to feel that it does its job well; the service provided should be demonstrated. The benefit of demonstrating good care is a boost for a practice team's morale, enabling it to feel valued and valuable. Case Study 7 shows how such an audit can be done simply, by using a 'tracer' condition (*see* Chapter 7).

Those who are against the demonstration of good care argue that it deflects energy from problems where there is considerable scope for improvement. However, if audit is always focussed upon things that appear to be wrong, it can have a depressing effect; a practice team is probably best served by attempting to achieve a balance.

Meeting patients' needs and expectations

Meeting patients' needs and expectations is properly two subjects.

1 The task of defining what patients need, and thereby being able to assess what their current health status is and how it might be improved.

2 The determination of what health care patients want, and whether they are satisfied with the health care they receive.

Determining the health status of a practice population is complicated, but increasing numbers of practices are defining risk factors and using these to determine who is at risk of certain conditions. The routine recording of weight (or body mass index), and current smoking, alcohol and dietary habits, are steps along the road to improving health status by reducing risk, especially for those diseases for which these are important aetiological factors.

By focussing on a single high risk factor, such as smoking, practices can identify those at increased risk by age and sex; these data can then be used to target preventive measures efficiently and thereby alter behaviour patterns to decrease risk. The use of audit in this way, for selecting, targeting and subsequently measuring change in patients' behaviour after an educational intervention, is a good example of how a practice can begin to improve the collective health of the people registered with it.

Finding out what patients want and expect from their general practitioners is a relatively new exercise in the United Kingdom. Surveys of patient expectations and satisfaction can lead to the identification of patterns from which standards can be formulated (*see* Example 2.9 and Case Study 3).

Example 2.9

The advice of patients was sought about the process of obtaining repeat prescriptions. Open-ended questions were asked and resulted in some unexpected answers. For instance, patients revealed that they would prefer not to come to the surgery for a repeat prescription, but would rather have their prescription sent to them in a stamped addressed envelope which they were prepared to supply.

Stimulating education

Doctors often cite the educational value of audit above any other. It can benefit a practice in several ways.

1 The value to the individual practitioner of feedback on personal performance. A doctor or nurse given access to the results of some aspect of their performance can more readily identify gaps in knowledge and skill, and so seek to remedy them.

2 The stimulus to learning when a group of partners or a primary care team review their current practice, with the objective of formulating new

criteria and standards for care, or of revising existing ones. Working together in this way combines educational benefit with the knowledge that the product, in terms of both skills and standards, will benefit the patients directly. Members of the practices involved in the audits described in this Chapter and Section II of the book would certainly attest to this. Several of the case studies (1, 4, 8, 10 and 13), revealed additional learning potential and needs within the practice team.

3 The generation of standards by a peer group, or the assessment of the results and the implications of audits carried out on each other. Standard setting and audit groups are growing in popularity; they have the added benefit of introducing new ideas from outside the practice.

In summary, there is a direct link between education and audit, which is most worthwhile when improved knowledge and skill leads to better patient care.

Promoting higher standards of hospital and community care

Consciousness of the quality of care in a general practice should make the practice team conscious of the quality of care given by other professionals to whom patients may be referred. In the near future, audit will extend to the assessment and evaluation of care given by hospital consultants, and workers in the community services. Practices should be prepared to make their own assessments and, where appropriate, specify their own standards for such services. Questions that could be addressed are shown in Box 2.4.

Box 2.4

- Are the waiting times for hospital outpatient appointments acceptable?
- What are the complication rates of particular types of surgery?
- What is the standard a practice specifies for access to diagnostic radiology or the laboratory?
- Are the consultants to whom patients are referred kind and considerate?
- Which groups of patients are attending follow-up clinics unnecessarily?

This extension of audit can open up the relationship between a general practice and its services, and can help to establish the practice as the patient's guardian and advocate in obtaining secondary care of good quality.

Bidding for resources

Within medical care, the competition for available resources is keener than ever, which means that practices must be able to demonstrate the range, quality and cost of their services. The ability to attract money for new services, or resources for the improvement of existing services, will be heavily dependent on the professionalism of the practice team. Similarly, effective quality assurance incorporating audit will be important in securing funds for the introduction of new ideas and technology to help develop the practice.

Effective defence

Audit and quality assurance are prerequisites for effective medical defence. In the UK hitherto, there has been only limited litigation against doctors, but this pattern may be changing. The regular use of audit should reduce risk by allowing a practice team to identify and eliminate areas of potential hazard before a mistake is made. The potential cost of medical defence to a practice may stimulate participation in risk avoidance procedures of which audit is the most important.

Summary

Although the benefits of audit discussed in this chapter are not comprehensive, they illustrate powerful and compelling reasons why the modern general practice should cultivate an interest in and knowledge of audit, building it into the regular routines of practice activity. The overall benefit is the stimulus audit can provide for all those concerned with the care of patients to seek and achieve improvement, by examining and questioning their professional practice, and by requiring the justification of the results of their care.

3 What is Audit?

Definitions

AUDIT, as defined in Chapter 1, is the 'method used by health professionals to assess, evaluate and improve the care of patients in a systematic way, to enhance their health and quality of life'. It consists of four basic steps which are summarized in Box 3.1 and shown in Fig. 3.1.

Box 3.1: Steps in audit

1 Identifying or defining criteria and standards, in order to answer the question 'What are we trying to achieve for our patients?'
2 Collecting data on current performance, i.e. the care given and its effects on patients.
3 Assessing performance against criteria and standards to determine the extent to which criteria and standards have been met.
4 Identifying the need for change, either to the way care is provided or to the criteria and standards.

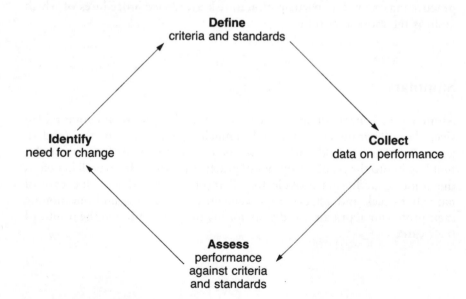

Figure 3.1   The audit cycle

This process of setting criteria and standards, monitoring performance, and identifying and initiating appropriate change is known as the audit cycle; it can be repeated as necessary to ensure progressive improvement.

The characteristics of audit as described above are found in most modern definitions (*see* Box 3.2).

Box 3.2: Some definitions of audit

1 The Quality Initiative of the Royal College of General Practitioners (RCGP, 1985)[1] asked doctors to:

- specify the services they provide;
- define objectives for patient care;
- assess their performance against these objectives;
- and, where appropriate, change clinical practice.

2 The Department of Health (DoH) White Paper *Working for Patients* (1989)[2] defined medical audit as:
'the systematic, critical analysis of the quality of medical care, including the procedures used for diagnosis and treatment, the use of resources, and the resulting outcome and quality of life for the patient'.

3 Shaw and Costain (1989)[3] described medical audit as:
'a systematic approach to the peer review of medical care in order to identify opportunities for improvement and provide a mechanism for realising them'.

4 Hughes and Humphrey (1990)[4] summarized the essential features of audit in general practice as:

- defining standards, criteria, targets or protocols for good practice against which performance can be compared;
- systematic gathering of objective evidence about performance;
- comparing results against standards and/or among peers;
- identifying deficiencies and taking action to remedy them;
- monitoring the effects of action on quality.

The term 'audit' is frequently used as a synonym for 'quality assessment' or 'quality assurance'. Quality assessment describes the monitoring and appraisal of care against predetermined standards. Quality assurance requires action to be taken on any deficiencies revealed by quality assessment. Audit that requires change is therefore comparable with quality assurance and contributes to it.

The value of questioning and justification

Audit stimulates doctors to ask questions about their work, to justify their actions to themselves and to their colleagues, and to modify their performance when necessary.

The examples of audit given in Chapter 2 and in the case studies suggest that 'auditors' should have a questioning frame of mind:

- What went wrong?
- Could we have done better?
- What does quality mean for this patient?

Self-questioning is a characteristic possessed by most professional people which ensures that they have appropriate knowledge and skills, and are effective. It requires self-discipline, and is best carried out in the company of working colleagues so that each individual may be stimulated by interaction.

The practice team who make time to question their direction, values, and specific aspects of care will welcome audit. A questioning attitude will help to define a team's objectives and standards, bring about change, and explore new ground.

The principle of justification is equally central to the practice of medicine.

- Can I justify the treatment I ordered for this patient?
- I think I should have seen that baby last night; can I then justify having given advice over the telephone?

In ordinary life clinicians tend to follow accepted patterns of 'good practice', for example, in establishing a diagnosis, or in organizing care. However, owing to a lack of sufficient time to reflect on every decision, significant departures from accepted patterns of practice should be justified; audit can provide data which might explain what happened and why.

A framework for assessing care

Audit requires a framework in which the description, measurement, comparison and evaluation of the quality of health care can be made. Avedis Donabedian (1966)[5] proposed that the quality of health care be regarded as comprising three interrelated parts, called structure, process and outcome. These three constituents of quality are shown in Fig. 3.2.

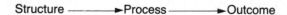

Structure ——————▶Process ——————▶Outcome

Figure 3.2   A framework for assessing care

Structure

The term 'structure' describes the physical attributes of health care, such as the surgery building, practice equipment, the number and kind of people in the practice team, and the patient records. Commonsense suggests that health care is likely to be more effective if it is carried out in comfortable surroundings with the right equipment and by the most appropriate people.

Although the presence of desirable structural attributes does not of itself ensure that the individual doctor or nurse will give good care, better care is more likely. For example, the doctors in a practice may have an electrocardiograph; its presence does not guarantee that they will use it appropriately, but if it was not present there would be no electrocardiograms to assist in the diagnosis. The absence of appropriate structure, such as in some practices situated in deprived areas, can diminish the chances of providing optimum care, even though competent doctors can give good care to some patients under adverse conditions. In other words, the structural features of a practice comprising the environment for care can promote quality or impede it.

The advantage of assessing the structural characteristics of care is that they are tangible and therefore can be counted thereby making audit easy. The earliest audit studies of British general practice were mainly concerned with structure. Audits were used most effectively in the new training practices of the 1970s to describe and assess such features as premises, equipment, staff and teaching facilities at a time when these varied widely. As a result, explicit criteria and standards governing the physical environment of teaching practices were laid down such that trainees could expect a consulting room of their own, a practice library with an appropriate collection of books and a basic order to patient records. These and similar standards can be re-audited to ensure that the practices involved in teaching young doctors are continuing to provide an environment most likely to facilitate learning.

Thus, the presence of structural attributes increases the chance of good quality care, but does not assure it. Structure, however, does not describe the performance of the health professional giving care; this is a fundamental weakness, and the reason why audits of structure are performed less often now.

Today, quality is assessed primarily on the basis of a doctor's performance. The performance of a health professional embodies Donabedian's two other constituents of quality — process and outcome.

Process

'Process' describes the care given by a practitioner, i.e. what the practitioner does, the sum of actions and decisions that describe a person's professional practice. Doctors and nurses tend to identify the process of care with quality because it describes what they do for their patients; it reflects their attitudes, knowledge and skill. Unlike structure, the process of care usually relates directly to the benefits patients derive as a result of care.

Studies of process, mainly of practice activity, may suggest better ways of doing things in the light of the most recent knowledge available. Audits of practice activities have investigated important aspects of care, such as prescribing habits, hospital referrals, laboratory and X-ray use, and patterns of clinical-decision making. Most of the case studies in Section II are process audits.

Outcome

Donabedian defined 'outcome' as the changes in a patient's current and future health status that can be attributed to antecedent health care. Outcomes are therefore the definitive indicators of health; they describe the effectiveness of care. For example, did the patient survive a potentially fatal condition, or were the effects of a potentially disabling condition prevented or alleviated?

Measures of outcome are more difficult to achieve than those of process, especially in general practice where so many conditions cannot be defined or diagnosed with precision. Some broad areas of outcome, decided upon by a consensus group of general practitioners, are shown in Box 3.3. These areas would have to be much more specific to become measurable entities.

Box 3.3: Measures of outcome

- Prevention of disease or control of the disease process.
- Improvement or preservation of the patient's level of function in the family, at work, and in social activities.
- Relief of the patient's symptoms, distress and anxiety, and avoidance of iatrogenic symptoms.
- Prevention of premature death.
- Minimizing the cost of the illness to patient and family.
- Patient satisfaction with care provided.
- Relief or clarification of the patient's interpersonal problems.
- Preserving the patient's integrity from an ethical point of view.

Source: Buck, Fry and Irvine (1974)[6]

In selecting outcome measures, the natural history of the disease has to be taken into account. For example, the care given to a patient with a minor virus infection would not be worth assessing because the condition is self-limiting — the outcome is predetermined and not related to any care given. Furthermore, the outcomes of chronic disease may not be apparent for many years, in which case it may be difficult to determine the contribution that care has made to outcome when compared with the many other factors that could have had an effect.

Intermediate outcomes

Much time and energy has been spent in arguing the relative validity, reliability, feasibility and cost of process and outcome measures as expressions of the quality of health care. Good measures of outcome are difficult to identify because it is hard to distinguish between the effects of antecedent care and other factors that may have influenced the patient's condition; the length of time that may have elapsed between giving care and its effects on the patient can also distort the suitability of outcome measures. Process measures are more suitable because they are immediate and easier to quantify; however, there is not always a causal relationship between care given (process) and the effects on the patient (outcome). For example, the prescription of the appropriate antibiotic (process) may be expected to shorten the period of disability (outcome) caused by a urinary tract infection; on the other hand, there is no good evidence to suggest that the use of cervical traction, manipulation or collar (process) is any better than placebo in altering the effects (outcome) of cervical spondylosis.

The term 'intermediate outcome' is used to describe measures that lie between true process and definitive outcome. The value of intermediate outcomes is that they are easier to measure yet they predict, or are assumed to predict, definitive outcome. For example, the immunization rate is the sum of each injection given (process), which is easy to measure, yet it has an excellent predictive value because it is known that a high immunization rate will prevent or severely restrict (outcome) the diseases against which protection is being given. Thus, the immunization rate can be used as a proxy for a definitive outcome. In this situation, it is unnecessary to wait for what could be years for definitive measures of outcome, such as the number of cases of infection that would ultimately occur in the immunized population, and the deaths or permanent disability that may result.

Audits of structure, process and outcome

Donabedian's framework for assessing quality defines one of the major parameters for describing audit. Thus, an audit of structure indicates an audit designed principally to assess the quality of the environment in which care is provided. A process audit describes the quality of work done by health professionals and an audit of outcome will assess the benefits achieved for patients. It is possible to design an audit that will assess all three aspects of quality. However, audits that assess the performance of the individual clinician or the practice team, which is what people are primarily interested in, will investigate a combination of process and outcome. Several of the case studies illustrate audits of process and intermediate outcome.

Summary

This chapter has defined audit and described three characteristics of quality care — structure, process and outcome. The audit approach can be applied to any or all of these, using methods which are described in Chapters 7 and 8.

4 Who Does Audit?

AUDIT can be performed by individuals (doctor, nurse, or other health professional) or a practice team who are investigating their own care (self-audit); there can be an audit of peers or an audit carried out by others external to the health professionals concerned (*see* Box 4.1). The relationship between the types of audit and the questions asked in the audit cycle (Fig. 3.1) are shown in Fig. 4.1.

Box 4.1: Types of audit

- Self-audit.
- Peer audit.
- External audit.

Self-audit

The term 'self-audit' is self explanatory. As said in the previous chapter, it is in the nature of professions that professional people should regularly question their own work and justify their actions to themselves. In the context of general practice, self-audit helps individuals and practice teams to carry out their implied or stated intentions, and to determine whether to change their behaviour, i.e. their way of practicing.

Regular self-audit can be difficult to sustain, often because other activities in a practice may claim priority. Owing to the immediate demands of patient care, and those of running the practice, audit may be an exercise for which the practice team will not have time; audit may be performed only when there is an enthusiast in the practice who will organize it and carry it out, invariably on a subject of his or her own choice. It is only if a practice team decide the benefits of self-audit (*see* Chapter 2) are important or necessary, that resources — time, space, money, skills — will be allocated to it regularly.

Self-audit is fundamental to good care. However, the main advantage and disadvantage of self-audit are related to the same factor — it is private within a practice. As an advantage, it offers the opportunity for frank discussion especially where things have gone wrong or where resulting changes may be disturbing for some members. As a disadvantage, it is easy

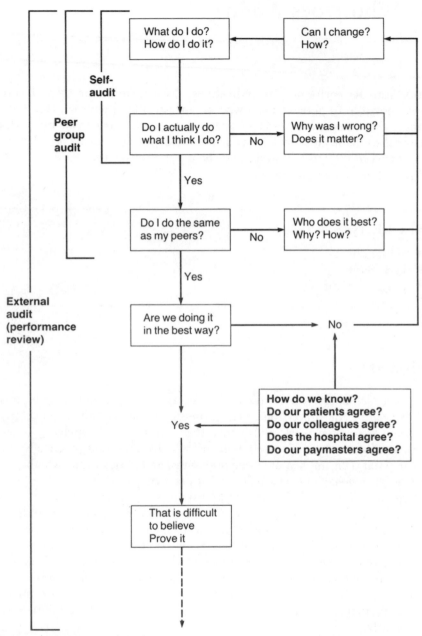

Source: Thornham R (1990)[1]

Figure 4.1 The relationship between the types of audit and the questions asked in the audit cycle

for the members of a practice team to collude and avoid awkward questions instead looking at areas that seem safe.

Peer audit

A peer is a person who is equal in any stated respect. In the context of audit in medicine, the word applies to a person in the same speciality or branch of medicine who has comparable experience and training. All principals in general practice are regarded as peers; trainees, although doctors working in general practice, would constitute a separate peer group.

When medical audit was first introduced in the USA in the 1930s, it was based on the principle of a review carried out by a doctor's peers. 'It takes one to know one' was the thinking behind this approach. In British general practice, peer review was introduced through vocational training. Today, it is usual for groups of trainees to meet to review case notes together. Trainer workshops operate on the peer principle when reviewing performance (*see* Example 4.1), and the national and regional structure and arrangements for selecting and re-selecting trainers are based on the principles of peer review. Peer groups in general practice tend to be local and concerned with items of mutual interest to members.

Example 4.1

The first trainer audit group in the Northern Region, which was set up in 1975, attempted to set criteria and standards for the care of patients with hypertension, enuresis and urinary tract infections. Two members of the group also scrutinized the records of each of the trainer's patients who died; selected cases were later discussed by the group. In addition, the group paid particular attention to the standard of their clinical record-keeping, especially as their first audit of a selected sample of records had shown how wide the gap was between intention and reality.

Source: Ashton et al., (1976)[2]

Local peer groups are ideal for generating inter-practice criteria and standards. For example, in the mid-1980s, most Northern Region trainers took part in peer group standard setting for common conditions in childhood.[3] Recently, similar peer groups of general practitioners in the Netherlands[4] met to consider criteria and standards that had already been formulated by experts. Both approaches have their place in audit by peer review in general practice.

One of the strengths of peer audit is that it is performed by colleagues in the same field of medicine; in many respects, it is general practitioners who are best placed to understand the possibilities and limitations of their discipline. Peer audit, therefore, is likely to be appropriate in context and as such, acceptable to colleagues.

The principal criticism of peer review is that it may become collusive. It is common for peers to recognise their own shortcomings in clinical practice when faced with the shortcomings of others during audit. For example, most practitioners are familiar with situations such as not writing up the case notes of patients seen at home, or prescribing penicillin indiscriminately for all sore throats. Because all practices are guilty of such shortfalls from time to time, especially when under pressure, they may not be examined as rigorously as possible and thereby go uncorrected.

Peer review is more threatening than self-audit; it introduces peers from outside the practice to make an independent assessment. However, that threat is tempered by the knowledge that, at some stage, the performance of these auditors will also be assessed by similar standards in the future.

External audit

The key difference between external audit and self-audit or local peer group audit is that the auditors do not have their own performance assessed. The audit groups may comprise general practitioners from another part of the country, they may belong to another specialty or profession, or they may include lay representatives. Consequently, they may represent quite different interests, values and priorities to those of the health professionals being assessed.

External audit can be threatening because it introduces assessors who are relatively detached and who may have different standards. Recently, it has often been associated with health service management, but external audit has its roots firmly in the medical profession (see Examples 4.2 and 4.3).

In general practice, the best known example of external review is the system operated jointly by the regional postgraduate organizations and the Joint Committee on Postgraduate Training for General Practice (JCPTGP), to set and monitor standards for vocational training, particularly for teaching practices.[7] These external audits have an educational element. However, their main purpose is managerial to ensure that training practices deliver the quality of service that they have been contracted to, such that trainees obtain the maximum benefit from their experience. It is likely that

---

Example 4.2

The earliest and best known examples of external audit in the UK were the Confidential Enquiries into maternal and perinatal deaths carried out jointly by the Royal College of Obstetricians and Gynaecologists (RCOG) and epidemiologists. These audits involved a meticulous examination of the case notes of all women and infants who died; from these national data, risk factors were identified which led to changes in clinical practice. As a consequence, maternal mortality and perinatal mortality rates have fallen. Outcome has been improved.

Source: HMSO 1957[5] and 1960[6]

Example 4.3

More recently, the Royal College of Surgeons (RCS) and the Faculty of Anaesthetists have been examining perioperative deaths on a confidential basis. These enquiries have already pinpointed aspects of surgical practice which in some units are causing unnecessary morbidity or death.

Source: Buck *et al.*, (1987)[7]

---

the Medical Audit Advisory Groups (MAAGs) will function in a similar manner in relation to the Family Health Service Authorities (FHSAs), by stimulating practices to implement systems of self- and peer audit. Later, the MAAGs may carry out external reviews of subjects important to the public health, such as reducing the number of deaths from coronary heart disease by identifying and reducing the risk factors in each practice population.

External audit has the theoretical sense that should bring greater objectivity to the assessment of performance. It is the prime means by which any practice's standards and performance can be monitored against a national norm or regionally agreed standards of practice. It may offer the best opportunity of raising basic standards, and of identifying individual practices and health professionals who fall below that minimum. The disadvantages are that because it can be seen as threatening, it tends to provoke a defensive attitude from those whose performance is being assessed. Doctors may be tempted to find out what the minimum standard is, and comply with that only.

A combination

Experience suggests that all three forms of audit are desirable in judicious combination. Self-audit should be the foundation of any system of quality assurance that undergoes regular improvement. The practice team motivated to question and initiate change from within is most likely to provide the best care, and achieve the highest standards.

Peer review is local, cheap and can act as a source of new ideas. It is now accepted as a valuable educational method in general practice that can bring measured objectivity without being overthreatening.

External review also has its place especially in establishing minimum standards. Practices will make sure that they function well if they know there is to be an external audit, especially if incentives or sanctions are attached. For example, in future, FHSAs may be unlikely to invest beyond the minimum in practices that provide poor care, however that is defined.

It seems clear that the more a practice does to set and monitor its own standards, the less likely it is to be at risk from external review.

5 How to do it: Getting Started

THERE are two important steps to be taken when considering an audit.

1 Choosing the subject.
2 Working out a design most likely to achieve the desired objective.

Choosing a subject

Sometimes it can be surprisingly difficult to decide on a topic for audit. Some basic ground rules that can be used to help are shown in Box 5.1; these should always be considered before committing resources.

Box 5.1: Ground rules for choosing an audit subject

Any subject chosen for audit should be seen by the practice team as:

- likely to benefit patients;
- likely to benefit the practice;
- relevant to professional practice;
- relevant to professional development;
- significant or serious in terms of the process and outcomes of patient care;
- having potential for improvement;
- capable of holding the interest and involvement of team members;
- likely to repay the investment of time, money and effort involved.

These guiding principles ensure that the subject chosen is meaningful to those professionals whose care is being audited.

Audit is often challenging; some members of the practice may have misgivings about their involvement in the process. For those who are unsure of the value of audit, the least that is required is a demonstration of the benefits (described in Chapter 2), and the chosen subject should be relevant. For practices in the early stages of learning about audit, careful attention to the choice will pay dividends in the form of involvement, if not commitment, from colleagues who may have a healthy cynicism towards this major shift in general practice.

Sources of ideas

The most obvious way of identifying a subject is through the trigger of a significant or adverse event in a practice, for instance, a patient complaint about treatment as illustrated in Case Study 11 or the premature death of a patient through a treatable cause, such as acute asthma, meningitis or hypertension as in Case Study 7.

Topics may arise as a result of a regular review either within or from outside the practice. Thus, practices who collect routine statistics might identify problems relating to prolonged waiting times for appointments, the failure of certain patients with diabetes to attend for reviews as in Case Studies 12 and 15 or an immunization programme (*see* Case Studies 5 and 14). Similarly, questions that need to be explored further may arise as a consequence of an external review, for example, when a peer group reviews the practice following an MAAG visit, or after a review of a teaching practice by the regional education committee for general practice.

Another source is the individual within a practice who has a particular idea that he or she wishes to pursue (as with the trainee in Case study 13). Most audits in general practice start in this way. These individuals will have particular priorities, which take precedence over other issues. Some of these ideas make a valuable place to start, although the 'bee in the bonnet' syndrome can be a diversion. Audit topics do have to be relevant to other team members.

Making the selection

There are several different sources of ideas for audit. These need to be brought together in the practice. A practice which has a philosophy of questioning and justifying as part of its ethos is likely also to have the sort of approach to management described in Chapter 10, and which is based on planning ahead and on documenting wherever possible where it stands at present. Such practices are likely to have some arrangement for prioritizing activities, including the selection of subjects for audit.

The selection of a topic for audit is likely to be made by the partners or the practice team in the context of a practice's overall development plan. It is important that the team has some criteria for making a rational choice. The general principles described in Box 5.1 provide a useful guide. Baker and Presley (1990)[1] list a series of questions that can also be applied (Box 5.2).

It is desirable that one member of the practice team should assume responsibility for keeping the candidate subjects for audit under review. Otherwise topics will be forgotten or the process of choice will become

---

Box 5.2: Questions to consider when choosing priorities

- Is the problem common?
- Does it affect patient care?
- Does it have serious consequences in terms of morbidity or mortality?
- Can it be solved using audit?
- Is it a management problem rather than one of audit?
- Is it a FHSA/DHA problem rather than one of the practice?
- Would correcting the problem save more money than ignoring it?
- Does the team have the skill to perform the audit?
- Does the team feel motivated to tackle the problem?

Source: Baker and Presley, 1990[1]

---

haphazard. It is a function of practice management to assign such responsibility.

Planning an audit

When setting out along the audit route it is often unclear quite what the process will be, or what methods are to be used and what resources are required. Unless considerable thought is given to these issues, it is quite possible to be precipitated into a data collection exercise only to discover, too late, that insufficient attention to the basic design casts doubt at a later stage on the viability of the project. It is not uncommon to find data being collected in a practice (often more than is needed for the purpose) that will not provide an answer to the question(s) being asked, or that are incompatible with data from other practices against which comparisons are to be made.

Failures in the execution of an audit demoralize the auditor, diminish the confidence of other team members whose care is being audited, and waste resources.

The key lies in thorough planning. Just as the practice as a whole is more likely to succeed if it identifies clearly where it wants to go and how to get there — the link with practice management again — so an audit is most likely to succeed if the same steps are followed. The most important of these are summarized in Box 5.3.

Box 5.3: Planning an audit: 10 guidelines

1 Define the nature of the perceived problem.
2 Produce a clear written statement of aims.
3 Select the most appropriate methods.
4 Decide upon other basic design features.
5 Identify the main analysis to be made.
6 State who the audit will involve.
7 Start small.
8 Have a short time-scale.
9 Proceed step by step.
10 Indicate how the possible need for change is to be handled.

---

1 Defining the problem. A general statement on the subject for audit should be followed by further definition of the perceived problem. Case Study 1 shows the value of this. For example, if the problem is one of managing asthma in children, the next question might focus on a specific aspect, such as early diagnosis, care during acute attacks, parental information or preventive therapy. Further definition is important, both for deciding the aims and choosing the methods.

2 Statement of aims. It is worth spending time achieving agreement in the practice on written aims, that are unambiguous and capable of being tested. The process of refining the aims will be facilitated by the discussion, in particular, the attempts to explain what the audit is about and what it should accomplish.

3 Choosing the method. Once the aims are clear, the method can be chosen. The choice will be influenced partly by appropriateness and partly by the availability of relevant resources. Chapter 7 gives details of the methods available.

4 Design decisions. It is important to decide whether the audit is to be confined to the practice, or whether others should be involved in some way, and, if so, what the consequences will be. The design may include provision for an intervention to be tested; in this case, data should be collected before and after the intervention so that change can be measured. Questions whether the audit should be retrospective or prospective, or whether sampling should be employed, are important and discussed in greater detail below.

Retrospective and prospective audits. Retrospective audits have the advantage that they can provide information quickly about the nature of care that has been given in the immediate past. Their weakness is that they are wholly dependent on the completeness of the clinical notes kept in the patients record, and good practitoners do not make clinical notes with the needs of some future auditor in mind. Retrospective clinical audits are better suited to the examination of the care of patients with chronic illness than that for those who have acute problems, because key events in the progress of a chronic condition are more likely to have been recorded.

Prospective audits look forward and are planned, with the aim of collecting data in a particular manner. Their strength is that the data collected are likely to give an accurate picture of the care the auditor wants to describe, provided that the method of data collection has been designed appropriately. One disadvantage of prospective audits is that they can alert the clinicians, whose performance is to be audited, to be on the lookout for what is expected of them and so alter their behaviour, which in unaudited circumstances might have been different.

Another variant is the audit that provides a 'snapshot' of the practice at a given point in time. Like other audits, they provide an opportunity to determine if pre-existing criteria and standards are being adhered to or to provoke further exploration.

Sampling. The technique of sampling enables the auditor to limit the amount of data collected without diminishing its value, especially its representativeness. Provided that the minimum number of cases to be examined during the audit is known, and also the number of cases seen during the audit period, it is possible to make best use of time by collecting data on only a proportion of cases.

Such an approach depends upon the study area, the number of cases presenting and the time over which data is to be collected. In a large practice with 200–300 known cases of diabetes, it may not be necessary to capture data on every case to answer the questions asked. By choosing to audit only a proportion of those cases, valid answers may still be reached, whilst saving time and effort. Sampling is simple provided that the whole population from which the sample is drawn can be identified. The care of diabetes provides a good example (*see* Example 5.1).

Drawing a random sample used to be done with random number tables — the more romantic enthusiasts then used such devices as the DOH lottery number generator. Today the random number function on any calculator suitable for GCSE mathematics is the nearest source to hand. This method is appropriate for general practice audit; the cases identified probably represent a spectrum of the diabetic illness within the practice.

A simpler method, known as systematic sampling, involves choosing a proportion of cases, for example, 10% by identifying every tenth case

---

Example 5.1

A practice wished to collect information about the compliance of patients with diabetes with dietary advice following a drive in the practice to improve this. The first step was to decide how many patient records should be examined to ensure representativeness. This was calculated to be 70 of a total population of 200 patients with diabetes (who were numbered). The second step was to generate a random set of numbers between 1 and 200 until 70 cases were identified.

---

on a register; the first case is chosen at random, for instance, number 7 on the register, the next case is 17 and then 27, and so on. However, a filing system in which patients are grouped by address can introduce bias into this sampling method.

Practices who require a more sophisticated approach to sampling are advised to consult the statistician at the DHA or specialists in the local department of public health. There is also an excellent chapter by Russell and Russell (1990)[2] which describes the statistical analyses for audit in general practice.

5 Analysis. As part of the design of the audit, it often helps to decide upon the main analyses to be made and even to rough out the shape further by drawing up draft tables. The purpose is not to anticipate the results, but to generate an appropriate design. In larger audits, this process might involve the use of a pilot audit to test the proposed design and method.

6 Who is involved? In a subject as sensitive as audit, it is important to write down who is to be involved, to ensure that everyone is aware and can make the appropriate commitment. This active participation should also ensure commitment to any of the changes found to be necessary after audit.

7–9 Step by step. The principles of starting small, and proceeding step by step over a short timescale are virtually self-evident. They set clear limits within which the audit takes place. These points need emphasizing because many auditors are easily carried away by their own enthusiasm.

10 Managing change. It is useful to have some idea about how the results are to be managed, especially if difficulties are expected; for example, the results could be critical of a particular individual. The ease with which this stage is handled will depend to a large extent on the professionalism of the practice's management systems (*see* Chapter 10).

The use of resources

It is important to decide on the maximum level of resources a practice team is prepared to commit to an audit. In doing this, it is also important to ensure that the subject examined is appropriate to the skills and resources available. Resources can be divided into several categories: time, money, people. Time is usually a limited resource; if staff are undertaking an audit, they are probably not able to perform another activity — known in economics as an opportunity cost. Although money can be used to buy more time, there is also an opportunity cost associated with this strategy. The original decision need not be rigid and it is almost inevitable that the required resources will be underestimated. Nevertheless an initial estimate of the available resources may help to determine the choices for such potentially expensive items as data collection.

The successful planning of an audit also includes continuous review. As each step of the audit becomes clear, the resources being used should be reassessed and compared with the original estimates, to ensure that the aims can be achieved. Regular checks are especially important if a practice team is performing more than one audit at a time, or the ongoing audit is part of regular performance monitoring. Audit has to be efficient, effective, give value for money, and contribute to the practice's overall purpose; it should not become an end in itself.

Summary

The emphasis in this chapter has been on the need for a planned approach to audit. Success is more likely to be achieved if early attention is given to aims that can be attained within the resources available.

6 How to do it: Criteria and Standards

THIS chapter describes the first step in the audit cycle (*see* Chapter 3), when the partners or the practice team identify their existing criteria and standards for patient care, or define new ones. Considering standards at the planning stage also helps to define the aims of the audit. This is not an easy subject. Yet without a clear understanding of the methods for setting standards, or their application in a clinical setting, audit is of limited value to a practice.

The first part of this chapter places criteria and standards in their clinical and operational context within the practice and describes their most important features. It concludes with practical suggestions about the process of setting standards within practices and peer groups.

The context

Doctors in any field of medicine work from a basis of 'good practice'. Good practice is the received wisdom of the day which indicates the best way of diagnosing or managing a patient's condition. It guides the decisions made by doctors about individual patients, and it is the yardstick against which a doctor's handling of a case may be judged, for example, by colleagues carrying out a peer review or in a court of law.

In its broadest sense, good practice is largely implicit. Implicit standards of good practice include for example comfort in the waiting room, courtesy, kindliness, a caring attitude and consideration for the feelings of relatives. The problem is that if standards remain implied, there is scope for misunderstanding and variation in their interpretation because they are subjective. Moreover, it is difficult to assess performance in an individual case against subjective, generally stated principles, and it is virtually impossible to make meaningful comparisons between groups of cases without explicit statements of expected performance.

There is a growing trend in medicine to overcome the problem of subjective standards by seeking to use explicit written statements, which are objective, and describe the care expected, and the level or standard it is desirable to achieve. The value of this approach is that it encourages the health professional to think more clearly about what should be accomplished in a way that will lend itself to subsequent measurement and assessment. Explicit, objective statements can be communicated easily to other team members, such that the chances of misunderstanding are reduced and individuals will find it easier to comply with what has been agreed. Explicit statements are also essential as the foundation for valid comparisons between practices.

The major disadvantage of explicit measurable statements is that there is a limit to what can be defined and measured in this way. The assessor may focus only on the measurable, and claim that only the measurable reflects quality. However, the attributes of care with implicit standards mentioned above are components of good quality care and have to be taken into account. Although explicit standards should be used wherever possible, the assessor should be prepared to make judgements on matters where standards can only be implicit.

Examples of practices working with simple explicit statements are given in Case Studies 4 and 15; in Case Studies 7 and 14, practice teams are trying to develop them. The audit cycle described in Chapter 3 begins with the stage of defining explicit statements describing criteria and standards for care; in Chapter 10, this process is directly related to that stage in the management cycle at which a practice team starts by defining its aims, objectives and standards for care. It may therefore be helpful to see in more detail what is meant by criteria and standards, and how they can be developed.

Criteria and standards

The term *criterion* is used to describe a definable and measurable item of health care which describes quality, and which can be used to assess it. Criteria are usually written in the form of statements that describe what should happen (*see* Example 6.1).

Example 6.1: Single statement criteria

- Females of susceptible age should be immunized against rubella.
- All children requesting attention for acute problems will be seen on the same day.
- Any patient will normally be offered a non-urgent appointment with any doctor within 48 hours, except in an epidemic.

A *standard* describes the level of care to be achieved for any particular criterion; continuing with the example of rubella immunization in Example 6.1, the standard might specify that 98% of the female population at risk should receive protection. The full criterion and standard are given in Example 6.2.

Example 6.2

- Females of susceptible age should be immunized against rubella (*criterion*).
- 98% of all females of susceptible age will be immunized against rubella (*standard*).

It may take practice to be able to make the distinction between criteria and standards. The best way to learn is to write out some simple statements similar to those illustrated in Examples 6.1 and 6.2.

There are many opportunities for using single statement criteria and standards of the kind illustrated above, in isolation. However, it is possible, through the careful selection of criteria, to build up a picture or map of the most important characteristics of a disease or a symptom. These aggregated criteria and standards describe good care.

Aggregated, explicit criteria and standards are being used increasingly in health care, including general practice; they are used to describe 'good practice' in the diagnosis and management of acute and chronic diseases and illnesses, in the management of preventive medicine, in the specification of patient access and for many organizational tasks. They can be assembled and presented as guidelines or protocols.

Guidelines or protocols can be presented as a series of statements or displayed in the form of a flow-chart, known as an algorithm. The algorithm has the advantage of showing the branched decision-making process and its options at each stage. Figs 6.1 and 6.2 are extracts from clinical algorithms used in general practice for the management of constipation and acute diarrhoea in children[1]. Further information about the construction and use of clinical algorithms in primary care is contained in the excellent paper by Schoenbaum and Gottlieb (1990)[2] and in the British Medical Journal series[3] of clinical algorithms.

As the care of many illnesses involves more than one member of the practice team, it is increasingly the case that the practice team, rather than the doctors alone, draw up explicit statements about the way that care should be given to certain groups of patients, and what the expectations of care are. Guidelines used for different purposes will require different degrees of detail and may be expressed in a variety of ways.

Content of criteria and standards

Criteria and standards can be further defined by the particular characteristic of care — structure, process or outcome — they are describing (*see* Fig. 6.3 for examples).

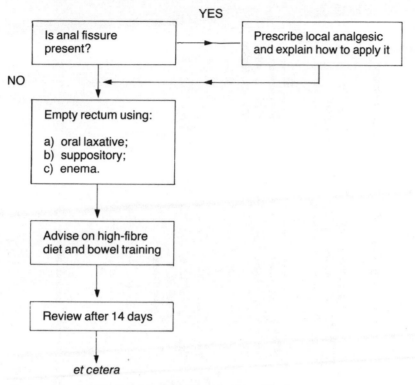

Source: North of England Study of Standards and Performance in General Practice
   (1990)[1]

Figure 6.1   An extract from the branching algorithm for management of constipation in
   children

Structural criteria and standards define aspects of the environment for
care. An example of a structural criterion indicating quality would be the
statement that:

'Patient record cards should contain a summary card'.

Continuing with this example, the structural standard, indicating the level
to be achieved, might be set at 50% initially; it could be raised as practice
teams reach this minimum standard, to ensure that improvement is maintained.

Process criteria and standards describe the care provided for the patient.
A process criterion might state, for example, that:

'The blood pressure for all patients aged 20–65 years should be taken and
recorded at least once every 5 years'.

Continuing with this example, a process standard would specify the

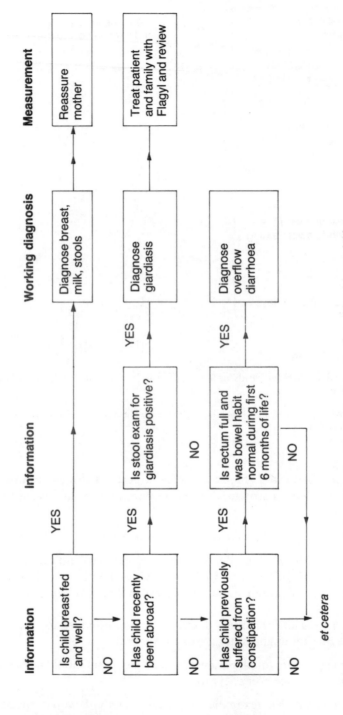

Figure 6.2　An extract from the branching algorithm for the diagnosis of acute diarrhoea in children

	Criterion	**Standards**
Structure	Patient records will include summary cards.	Should apply to 50% of records.
Process	All patients aged 20–65 years will have their blood pressure recorded in the notes at least once, within the last 5 years.	This should apply to: 50% of records in year 1, 75% of records in year 2, 95% of records in year 3, following the introduction of the standard.
Outcome	Patients with established hypertension aged 20–35 years will have a diastolic level less than 90 mmHg within the first year of treatment.	The target level will be achieved in 80% of cases.

Figure 6.3   Examples of criteria and standards

frequency with which the criterion should be achieved, for instance, in the first, second and third years following the introduction of this particular criterion.

Criteria and standards of outcome describe the effects of care on the patient. Continuing with the example about blood pressure, an outcome criterion might state that:

'In young adult patients with hypertension a diastolic pressure of 90 mmHg or less should be achieved within 1 year of commencing treatment'.

The standard of outcome might require that 80% of such patients should achieve the criterion within the stated period.

In distinguishing between *process criteria and standards* and *criteria and standards of outcome*, it is important to remember that *process criteria* describe the care given and *outcome criteria* describe the effects on the patient. Better process does not always result in better outcome. For example, a practice team could give assiduous attention to the process criteria and standards for blood pressure described above, making sure that blood pressure was measured and recorded in the notes to the standard required. They might be tempted to conclude that the patients were benefiting from this carefully regulated care. In fact, patients would benefit only if the practice team were able to show that the blood pressure level was controlled satisfactorily in accordance with the standard of outcome set. Were that not to be the case the only evidence of quality would be the frequency with which blood pressure measurements appeared in the notes. This distinction is nicely illustrated in Case Study 15.

Level of standards

There is always controversy when decisions have to be made about the precise level at which a standard should be pitched. There are three options basically, all of which can be illustrated using current standards for mumps, measles and rubella (MMR) immunizations in children under the age of 2 years.

A *minimum* standard describes the lowest acceptable standard of performance. Minimum standards are often used to distinguish between acceptable and unacceptable practice. For example, the Department of Health (DoH) has defined its minimum standard for immunization in the New Contract as at least 70% of all children eligible. The DoH underlines the use of this standard to define what it considers to be the boundary between acceptable and unacceptable practice by not making a bonus payment for any immunization programme that fails to reach the 70% target.

An *ideal* standard describes the care it should be possible to give under ideal conditions, when there are no constraints on resources of any kind. An ideal standard almost by definition cannot be attained. Continuing with the example, an ideal standard would require that *all* children within a practice would have completed a course of immunization by 2 years.

An *optimum* standard lies between the minimum and the ideal. Setting an optimum standard requires a judgement to be made about the best balance between, for example, the outcome for the individual patient and equity for patients as a whole in terms of resources available. Optimum standards represent the standard of care most likely to be achieved under their normal conditions of practice. They are most likely to reflect the good practice any conscientious general practitioner could be expected to achieve. The DoH definition of the 'optimum' standard for childhood immunization is a 90% immunization rate of those eligible. To reinforce the attainment of this standard, the DoH gives a higher payment for all practice immunization programmes that reach or exceed the optimum standard.

The derivation of criteria and standards

Criteria and standards can be derived from either the most recent medical literature and the best experience of clinical practice, or current societal and professional values — 'normative' criteria. Criteria can also reflect patterns of care taken from existing data and thereby current practice — 'empirical' criteria. In some ways, empirical standards are weaker than those drawn from the 'state of the art', precisely because they are a reflection of statistical averages which might or might not reflect good care.

For a practice considering defining criteria and standards for the first time, a combination of the two is best. It is worthwhile taking current patterns of care into account; but these should be set in the context of what it is best to do in terms either of the science of medicine or of the values of society and the health professions.

Internal and external standards

Another way of looking at criteria and standards is to consider who sets them. There are two options — internal or external. Internal criteria and standards are determined and set by practitioners whose care is subsequently assessed by audit. In effect, the individual practitioner, the practice team (comparable to self-audit) or possibly the local peer group set the criteria. The advantage of internally determined standards is ownership; doctors who have created their own standards will be motivated to implement the product of their own work.

External criteria and standards are created by any individual or group who is not being assessed. The advantage of externally generated criteria and standards is that they are likely to be more rigorous in their construction. The disadvantage is that they may have to be imposed; if so, those whose care is to be assessed may question them and be grudging in their willingness to implement and maintain them.

The solution lies in a balance between internal and external criteria and standards. A practice team should construct and use internal working clinical standards for everyday practice wherever possible, so that its members can see what they are trying to do and what they actually achieve. National external standards should be used selectively; few areas in medicine lend themselves to dogmatic statements that cannot be challenged.

In between, there is considerable scope for the implementation of local external working standards, which might be determined by a local group of doctors and nurses who want to determine the best care they can give in their district. Examples of locally agreed standards could include the care of patients with asthma, the early management of acute chest pain, and the ongoing care of patients with diabetes when it is shared between the general practice and hospital. This kind of initiative is likely to develop in future, as MAAGs and district audit committees begin to work together across the boundary between primary care and the hospital service.

Working on criteria, standards and guidelines

There are several points that should be borne in mind when constructing criteria, standards and guidelines. In particular, it is necessary to:

- make unambiguous statements;
- keep the task focussed on the audit topic;
- refer to the literature indicating current practice;
- choose criteria and standards in line with current practice;
- ensure that criteria and standards are based on fact.

Health professionals often fail to take account of the work of others. Referring to published work is essential to avoid the danger of making statements that are inaccurate. The librarian at a local postgraduate centre can provide invaluable help in identifying references.

A practice team should be open to using guidelines that have been developed by other clinicians. Although the team may wish to make certain adjustments, much time and effort can be saved by using previously constructed guidelines. Some useful examples are to be found in the RCGP clinical folders.[4]

It is often best to construct criteria, standards and guidelines in a group because interaction among individuals is likely to achieve a better result than that achieved by individuals working in isolation. Experience suggests that there are three specific factors that will facilitate the work of a group and thereby improve its chances of success.

1 At least one member of the group should be familiar with the literature on current practice. An expert may be invited to attend the group so that he or she can act as a clinical resource when necessary.
2 One member of the group should have had at least some experience in the technique of writing criteria and standards, and of translating these into workable guidelines or algorithms.
3 The group should have a good chairman. It is often difficult to be productive and achieve a consensus about what constitutes good care. A good chairman will help the group to get a good result while a leaderless group will get lost.

Summary

Once the basic technique for constructing criteria and standards has been learned and mastered, health professionals will find this activity stimulating and rewarding. If criteria and standards have developed within a practice, much will be learnt about what the members of a practice want; it is a valuable team-building exercise as well as a learning exercise. By concentrating on explicit criteria and standards wherever possible, a practice team will develop a series of statements about patient care it considers to be important and which reflects quality. This can then be used as the basis for subsequent audit or performance monitoring. Such statements can be revised and updated regularly.

7 How to do it: Data and Methods I

IN this chapter, the principal sources of data for audit in general practice are described. On occasion, data sources, data collection and audit methods can be considered to be equivalent, for example, in surveys and interviews. In other cases, e.g. medical records, the data may be used for more than one audit method i.e. as more than one data source. For simplicity, the methods for carrying out an audit that use more than one data source are described in Chapter 8.

Many practices now have computers and use them both for data storage and audit. This can make audit easier, particularly when dealing with larger amounts of data. However much audit can be done with simple data collection and analysis using manual methods.

Many audits start with data collection, and the first stage of the audit cycle, i.e. defining criteria and standards, is omitted. This is legitimate, especially if the purpose of the audit is to carry out a preliminary reconnaissance of some aspects of a practice team's work.

The eight most commonly used sources of data are shown in Box 7.1. Each data source will be described using a format that indicates the origin of the data, how the data can be collected, how the data can be used, and an assessment of its strengths and weaknesses.

Box 7.1: Data sources and data collection

- Routine practice data
- External data
- Medical records
- Practice activity analysis
- Prospective recording of specific data
- Surveys
- Interviews
- Direct observation

Routine practice data

Routine practice activity generates data that are often used for regular performance monitoring. These data are varied and may be quite detailed.

Source

Data that should be readily available are the records of practice claims to the FHSA. For example, every practice should have a record of immunizations carried out, cervical cytology examinations undertaken, hospital referrals made (from 1991), prescribing patterns (PACT), and night calls made between 10 pm and 8 am.

Many practices routinely keep other data to describe workload. For example, appointments and visiting books will show the number of patients consulting, the number of house calls made, the number of out-of-hours calls, the attendances at antenatal clinics, and the number of patients seen in the treatment room by the practice nurse.

Every practice also has basic registration data about patients that will indicate patients' age and sex, marital status and postcode. Some practices may have other registers, for example, a disease index, registers of certain age-groups — children under 5 years or patients over 75 years — or a register of the permanently housebound who live alone. Occupation may be recorded. Many practices also keep a record of the annual number of livebirths, stillbirths and terminations, and every practice has either the death certificate books or hospital correspondence which taken together can show who died and the registered cause of death.

Finally, the annual practice accounts contain data under the main headings of expenditure and income, from which financial trends may be detected.

How to collect the data

The first step is to recognize the potential value of data that practice teams record routinely in support of their management functions. These data should then be structured, such that the information is readily available and accessible. Then it is a matter of assembling the data using a simply designed data collection sheet or by entering the data into the practice computer directly. Results can be analysed either manually or using a basic computer programme (see also Chapter 9).

Uses

These data have four main uses.

1 Data may be used to control some practice activities. For example, a practice team intending to achieve the top target for immunization regularly will need to know who has been immunized, on a weekly basis. Case Studies 2 and 5 show data being used in this way. Similarly, routine

monitoring is used to control aspects of income and expenditure to ensure that all claims are made and cash flow is satisfactory.

2 Routine monitoring can alert a practice team to minor changes which, if allowed to continue over time, may become significant. For instance, an insidious increase in the interval that patients have to wait between requesting an appointment and being seen may be highlighted by routine monitoring, allowing remedial action to be taken before a crisis occurs and complaints are made.

3 Routine monitoring may chart the progress of a change in practice policy. For example, the impact of a practice decision to immunize all adults against tetanus can be monitored either through the number of prescriptions being claimed from the FHSA in non-computerized practices or from a practice's computer record.

4 Routinely collected data are used in several audit methods. For example, they should contribute to the overall profile of a practice which is built up during the course of a practice visit. In some practice activity analyses, they can act as substitutes for or complements to data that have to be collected specifically for an audit, which are more expensive.

Strengths and weaknesses

The great strength of these data is that they are cheap and easy to collect because they are derived from regular practice activity. If used to monitor performance, they have an additional value in that they can act as a trigger for more specific audits designed to explore certain aspects of performance in more detail. The weakness of these data is that they are limited in scope to a screening function and can contribute only marginally to other audits a practice may have in mind.

External data

As changes in the NHS gather pace, so too will the flood of data from external sources. Some of this will be information, i.e. data that has already been interpreted. More often, data will require analysis to transform it into information relevant to the context of general practice.

Source

The local FHSA and DHA are becoming the commonest sources of external data; some of these data may be the trigger for a practice audit. For example, the DHA collects detailed data on the workload and case-mix of community nurses and health visitors. These data describe a major aspect of care given to patients in a practice, and are relevant to a practice team trying to build a picture of practice activity.

The FHSA is now the best source of data on a practice's prescribing patterns. The PACT analysis and feedback indicate what is possible. Similar analyses and feedback can be expected shortly on patterns of referral to hospitals. FHSAs and DHAs are also becoming a source of non-routine data. For example, with computerization of the FHSA, it is possible to request specific analyses of the age–sex and geographical distribution of the practice population. The DHA could be asked to provide a breakdown of census data relating to the practice area.

How to collect the data

The main problem with health authority information is volume. The only practical strategy for handling large volumes of data is for the practice, as part of its management functions, to designate one person in the practice team to be responsible for reviewing a particular subject area regularly, and for reporting any matters of potential interest to the team. The practice should also have a mechanism for bringing data from widely disparate sources together to index them again as part of the practice's management systems.

Uses

The main benefit of data from external sources lies in its relevance to practice policy-making and in stimulating new initiatives. For example, a significant change in the FHSA quarterly returns on additions to or removals from the practice list may lead to a further audit designed to find out why. Improved feedback on immunization rates, cervical cytology screening, breast cancer screening, and the use of the X-ray and laboratory services by individual partners should stimulate regular discussions within the team, some of which may prompt a more detailed audit of some particular aspect. Detailed information of the type generated by PACT level 3 can provide the basis for a variety of future audits, as illustrated in Case Study 6. For instance, the implementation of an agreed practice policy for prescribing antibiotics can be monitored through PACT data with minimal effort for data collection, but not for data interpretation.

Strengths and weaknesses

As with the routine general practice data, the format of externally produced routine data is fixed and may not always be appropriate to the task. However, it is usually cheap (sometimes free) and can provide comparisons with other practices. DHAs and FHSAs hold increasingly effective data sets on health needs assessment. It is the responsibility of a practice team to find out what is available and make best use of it.

Data from medical records

Medical records in general practice vary widely in their structure and content, and therefore in their usefulness as an audit tool. Some practices have well-ordered records which give a reasonably clear and complete account of the care given to patients, containing summaries of significant events, showing current medication, and recording the clinical details in a common format. However, records can be disorganized with only a few clinical details recorded.

The medical record should be one of the most important sources of data, especially for retrospective clinical audit, because it is the account closest to direct observation and is a means of knowing what happened to any patient. However, the potential discrepancy between the case and the record will depend entirely on whether a practice has policies and standards for record-keeping that ensure a minimum content consistent with a coherent account of care given.

The introduction of the A4 record into general practice (not yet wide-spread other than in Scotland) has improved the standard of record-keeping and thereby the potential value of medical records for retrospective audit. The A4 record, by virtue of its structure and size, encourages a more consistent recording of clinical events and the data, such as summaries, prescriptions, and demographic details, are located in properly identified areas.

Computerized records provide a major opportunity to access data retrospectively because of the highly structured format of the record and the ability of an increasing number of computer programmes to search for selected data items.

How to collect the data

Records must be searched and the relevant data abstracted from the mass of other material. For paper records, this can be a tedious task because one can never be sure that the data sought actually exist without trawling through each individual record. This is not too difficult when only 20 to 30 records are involved, but it becomes substantial and time-consuming if 200–300 records are to be examined. Moreover, the data required may be held in different parts of the record, in the correspondence, or on the summary sheet for instance.

To make abstraction as simple as possible, clinical records should be well structured. It is particularly helpful if a common format is agreed among the practice team. The problem-orientated approach is one way; a useful variation of this is to use the following headings:

- Presumptive diagnosis
- Evidence for diagnosis
- Management decisions
- Reasons for management decisions

It is equally essential to have a well-structured audit recording sheet so that the data abstracted can be collected efficiently and accurately.

Data that has been computerized are *usually* easier to access than those from paper records, although some of the earlier software programmes offered frustratingly limited opportunities from what should be a rich data source.

Uses

Retrospective data collected from records can provide insights into previous clinical practice; more accurately, they can give insights into the aspects of clinical care that have been recorded. In Case Study 4, the patient record has been used in this way.

An examination of the patterns of previous care may indicate problems that require further explanation. It is usual to use a retrospective audit to identify a problem initially, which can be further examined using a prospective audit in which the clinicians are asked to record relevant data in a specifically structured, and therefore easily abstractable, form.

Strengths and weaknesses

The use of previously recorded data has the advantage of requiring only limited effort and it can be collected over a short time-scale. The 'quality' of the results depends partly on the overall standard of the records. If the records are unstructured and hand-written, the return may not reflect the effort required. However, if an extensive data set has been collected, retrospective data collection should always be considered as one of the data sources for a practice audit.

Practice activity analysis

Practice activity analysis (PAA) is the term used to describe the examination of patterns of care in general practice, particularly those actions that doctors undertake frequently, such as prescribing, using laboratory and X-ray facilities, and referring patients to hospital. It was one of the earliest audit methods introduced into general practice, beginning in 1975 with the pioneering service provided by Drs Crombie and Fleming at the Birmingham Research Unit of the Royal College of General Practitioners[1]. Practice activity analysis is relatively easy to design and carry out. It quantifies the major activities in general practice and thereby helps to build a picture of the work of a practice. There are two principal types of practice activity analysis: one relates to the activities of a single practice team; the other follows the model of the large-scale data collection from several practices of the kind described by the College.

For the individual practice, practice activity analysis is a form of structured data collection which is clearly formatted for audit purposes. Large-scale practice activity analysis involves contributions to a general pool of data to generate 'norms' against which any individual practice can be compared. Various agencies provide this service, the best known being the RCGP Birmingham Research Unit. However, as MAAGs become established, it is likely that they will provide such a service to practices in their area.

How to collect the data

A structured form is used to record a preselected set of data items (*see* Fig. 7.1). These data can be analysed easily within the practice on a computer using a spreadsheet programme or a database such as dBase III. Another option is to seek help from the DHA or FHSA information services manager.

Any member of the practice team can be involved in data collection — nursing and administrative staff are often more rigorous and accurate than doctors. Most often, however, the bulk of data collection will take place at the time of a consultation.

Uses

Practice activity analysis within a single practice can provide an overview of important aspects of a practice's function, such as use of laboratory and X-ray facilities or workload patterns. Regular and planned events are particularly suitable for this mode of analysis. They can be used to monitor

Patient characteristics		Case numbers								
		1	2	3	4	5	6	7	8	→
Patient > 60 years	1									
Owns own house	2									
Married	1									
Family history of diabetes	3									
Smokes 10+/day	1									
Uses insulin	2									

Key:
1 = Yes; 2 = No; 3 = Don't know/no response.

Figure 7.1   Practice activity analysis coding sheet

progress to previously agreed standards, or as the starting point for a more detailed audit of a particular aspect. The content of the data set needs to be defined with the required uses in mind; trawling randomly for chance events is unlikely to be efficient. Case Studies 1, 5 and 10 show the use of practice activity analysis.

Inter-practice comparisons can provide an interesting perspective on a practice's performance, and may influence the process of care in such areas as immunization. Because they can provide comparisons with a selected data set they can enable comparisons to be made of practices working in similar circumstances, or at least provide the information necessary to understand the reasons for any differences in those circumstances.

Strengths and weaknesses

Practice activity analysis has three major advantages.

1 It can provide a framework for identifying patterns of events which hitherto may have been hidden.

2 It furnishes direct comparisons with the performance of colleagues. Opportunities for external review, as part of peer review, may originate from this point.

3 It can be used as a prompt or trigger for more specific audits on areas of interest or concern.

Practice activity analysis has two possible weaknesses.

1 If there is a substantial commitment to data collection, which has to continue for a long time, the willingness of a practice team may evaporate and the accuracy of the data can be compromised.

2 Practice activity analysis is more suited to showing patterns and rates than it is at revealing the underlying reasons for such patterns. For example, although practice activity analysis of hospital referrals would disclose variations in patterns and rates, a specifically designed prospective audit would shed light on the decision-making processes of clinicians which account substantially for such variations in the first place.

Prospective recording of specific data

Many audits require the collection of a specific data set, comprising a number of data items not usually recorded or which need to be recorded in a particular format. In these circumstances, the data must be newly collected, either at a particular point in time, a cross-sectional study, or over a period of time, a longitudinal study. The definition of the items will have been refined through the process of planning the audit and formulating the clinical criteria and standards.

How to collect the data

One of the simplest methods of collecting specific data is to ask the health professional to record the required items at the appropriate time for example, when writing a prescription or making a referral or ordering an investigation. However, the clinician needs guidance to ensure that only the required items are collected, because every item collected adds time and effort to the consultation. Wherever possible, the items should be recorded on a computer, which will allow the rapid generation of aggregated data at the end of the collection period.

An alternative strategy is for the data collector to record the required items on audio tape, which can then be transcribed by a secretary onto a paper or computer record. This technique is particularly useful for data collection outside the surgery. The practice administrative staff might also collect some of the non-clinical material relevant to each case.

Uses

Audits of care for relatively frequent events are often well served by data set recording. Usually, these data relate to the process of care, i.e. the care provided by the professional during the consultation. An audit of prescribing patterns, for instance, which requires a data set of age, sex, presenting symptoms, working diagnosis, treatment and result, might necessitate the use of the prospective data collection method. Another example might be the planned monitoring of care for a particular group of patients who have a chronic condition, such as hypertension, asthma or recurrent urinary tract infection. An encounter form can be held in each patient's record for completion at the time of consultation. Case Study 2 gives an example of this.

Strengths and weaknesses

Data collection forms act as a prompt for the doctor or nurse. This prompt may distort the results of the audit, which may not have been as positive if there had been no such prompt. This effect can be overcome only with considerable effort, and for the purpose of operational practice audit the resulting lack of distortion is generally not worth the expenditure of effort. The minimum data set and recording system does require forethought which can assist in clarifying the purpose of the audit.

It is important to remember that a considerable amount of data can be collected by this method, not all of which can be used effectively.

Surveys

Many practices are only just discovering the value of the survey method as a valuable means of gathering information about the health of the practice population or about their expectations of its services. Essentially, surveys are a method of collecting data about some aspect of a patient's life by means of a questionnaire that the individual completes. Whichever method of survey is chosen, it is important to recognize the rules of survey methodology, and the practice team wishing to explore this method further will find it helpful to consult Abrahamson.[2] Time spent with this lively and concise work will save considerable effort — and potential disappointment — later.

Source

Surveys can be undertaken by post or on forms handed out in the surgery waiting room. The forms can vary from a relatively unstructured format in which the questions elicit a variety of written answers to a highly structured format in which the respondent ticks boxes. Surveys can be carried out on small or large numbers of people, different methods being used for various purposes. Surveys can be used to collect data about the process of care, the care patients receive, or the outcomes of care, including patient satisfaction. An increasing number of standardized questionnaires are commercially available, although care must be taken over choice. Case Study 3 demonstrates the use of a postal survey.

How to collect the data

Survey questionnaires are targeted at specific groups of people. The group may be identified by a particular characteristic, such as age or diabetes, or because they were engaged in a certain activity at a particular time, for instance, every woman who has attended an antenatal clinic in the past year, or every adult who has sat in the waiting room during the past month. The data can be used to perform a cross-sectional audit (that is, once only) or to review the process of care over time.

A record must be kept of who (or what numbers) receives the questionnaire, when and why. The practice age–sex register (computer or card index) may be used to identify recipients. This information is vital to understand the response rates and the context in which the data were collected.

Uses

A wide range of audits can be supported by survey methodology. Provided that the questionnaire has been properly designed, information on issues such as the outcome of care for chronic disease, patient satisfaction or morbidity can be collected.

Strengths and weaknesses

Surveys can produce a plethora of data unless appropriate thought has been give to data management and analysis. The use of sampling should always be considered to limit the data collected to that sufficient to satisfy the audit design (see Chapter 5). Surveys are also relatively costly in terms of production and postage (where necessary). If many people do not return the questionnaires, reminders will have to be sent. None of these hazards should dissuade a practice from considering surveys. Patients are often willing to provide information useful to their own health care or to improve the service they use, and surveys are a valuable way of achieving these ends.

Interviews

Information based on data collected by interviewers is usually more detailed than survey data, although the numbers of respondents is usually limited. Despite the fact that much data collection in primary health care is based on a particular type of interview, i.e. the consultation, it is relatively uncommon for the data for a general practice audit to be collected in this manner. There may be several reasons for this.

1 Interviews should be carefully structured (even if they are 'unstructured').
2 It is recognized that analysis is sometimes difficult.
3 Interviewers are often expensive to employ, which substantially increases the costs of an audit.

   Nevertheless, with careful attention to method, the selection of topics and techniques, interviews can prove to be a useful method of data collection for audit.

How to collect the data

The development of interview questionnaires and their analysis is well covered by Abrahamson[2]. A carefully worded questionnaire can elicit more detail about the health care and health status of an individual than any of the preceding methods. Although the answers may be translated into a coded form, the opportunity to select a certain feature and follow it through in depth is available. Additional comment can be recorded verbatim to illuminate the audit results, an important skill to be learned by those who use this method.

Uses

Complex or sensitive issues that cannot be addressed easily by methods such as postal questionnaires often lend themselves to investigation through interviews — for example, the effects of treatment, particularly if there are embarrassing side-effects, such as sexual dysfunction. Unusual or rare events may also be best investigated through the medium of the interview, e.g. the care provided for people who have a terminal illness for which a sensitive approach is essential, or an audit of adverse events, such as preventable death in people under 65 years of age. Aspects of the process and outcomes of care can be examined using this technique.

Strengths and Weaknesses

Interview technique is different from consultation techniques in general. Perhaps because of this doctors do not make the best interviewers. Some training in interview techniques is usually necessary to derive the most of this method. Consequently, it may be appropriate to 'buy-in' the necessary interviewing and analysing skills.

The major advantage of this method is its potential to provide insights into complex issues.

Direct observation

There are several ways in which the process of care can be audited using direct observation, although it is one of the most difficult methods to use and analyse successfully. The most obvious technique of direct observation is to have an observer in the consultation, although this invariably alters the dynamic being observed. Other techniques include direct observation through a 'one-way' mirror (now rather out of fashion), and audit and video recording. Some of these methods are regularly used for teaching in general practice, and have been advocated as a means of reviewing performance in the RCGP's 'What sort of doctor?'[3]

How to collect the data

The capture of raw data is difficult in direct observation. Problems occur when the observations have to be reduced to reproducible data, because any implicit judgements made about the data hold as much value as implicit criteria and standards for care.

Several techniques exist for analysing the content of consultations, many of which are complex and costly. If an audit has limited objectives, e.g. the aim is to record whether a doctor gives advice on stopping smoking to a smoker with a chest infection, a relatively simple data collection form will suffice; unfortunately, a mass of raw data, in the form of consultations, might have to be reviewed in order to achieve even this limited objective.

Uses

The process of care, inter-personal skills and specific types of information exchange can all be examined using direct observation. However, this method has more value in education than audit. For example, doctors who sit in on each other's consultations use this as an opportunity to learn from their colleague's best practice. Video consultations are also discussed among peers, which is a less challenging approach to reviewing clinical performance in individual cases.

Strengths and weaknesses

Direct observation allows the doctor/patient interaction to be investigated. Its use as a method of examining particular clinical problems is limited by the frequency of presentation, although this is not a constraint in audits of special sessions such as a diabetic clinic. The greatest constraints are the time it takes to observe and analyse the process of care, and the challenge of being observed by peers or experts. Paradoxically, that challenge is also one of the greatest strengths of this method.

On balance, the problems outweigh the advantages. Direct observation is used only infrequently in multi-case audit because of the complexity and cost of analysis.

8 How to do it: Data and Methods II

THIS chapter outlines those audit methods that make use of several sources of data. The main audit methods in general practice, including those already described in the previous chapter, are summarized in Box 8.1. The use of practice data for routine performance monitoring, practice activity analysis, surveys and interviews and direct observation have already been considered. There remain three important approaches to audit that involve the collection of data from more than one source.

Box 8.1: Audit methods

- Routine performance monitoring
- Practice activity analysis
- Surveys and interviews
- Direct observation

- Confidential enquiries
- Use of tracers
- Practice visiting

Confidential enquiries

The confidential enquiry is a method relatively new to general practice. There are two separate but complementary approaches.

1 *Single critical events*. The examination of single, critical events can be one of the most productive and effective forms of audit in general practice. This approach developed from the 'random' case analysis used for teaching vocational trainees. This teaching method has been formalized and refined, mainly by ensuring that the scope for enquiry is broadened beyond the clinical notes used in case analysis to include the direct questioning of all concerned with a particular situation, and also by adopting a structured format for writing down the findings and conclusions.

The examination of single critical events is concerned primarily with the reduction of clinical and organizational error, examples of which were described in Chapter 2. The aim of this method is to discover flaws in the process of care, the correction of which will have a beneficial effect on outcome for future patients.

A case study involving all the members of one family and all the partners of a practice is described in detail in Case Study 11. It may be helpful to read this case history at this point because it gives an indication of how such a situation can arise, how it can be investigated systematically, by drawing on both the case notes and interviews with the people concerned, and what changes can result. Another very graphic example is given in the *Who killed Susan Thompson?* video and course book from the RCGP.[1]

2 *Aggregated critical events.* The examination of aggregated clinical and organizational critical events is usually external. The approach was pioneered by the RCOG in the 1950s in their confidential enquiries into maternal and perinatal deaths[2,3], and by the RCS in the 1980s into perioperative deaths,[4] (*see* Chapter 4). This approach is now being introduced into general practice. For example, Northumberland District Health Authority[5] is currently enquiring into deaths from cervical cancer in women; an important part of this audit involves a detailed exploration of the screening process and of the events that may have led to a delay in the diagnosis in the setting of general practice. In future, aggregated data from critical incidents are likely to be collected and used by practices themselves. The choice of subject is important; the resources required to achieve a good result can be justified only if the error can be reduced significantly. Examples that fulfil this criterion include delay in the diagnosis of cases of meningitis, error in the treatment of an acute attack in asthmatic children, and the inappropriate management of acute chest pain.

Method

As the use of this method is wholly dependent on confidence and trust, it is essential that every member of a practice team who may become involved agrees to the audit *before* a single case is examined. Critical incidents and events are liable to reflect badly on certain individuals; careless handling of audit can cause offence, damage confidence or result in non-cooperation.

The confidential enquiry is likely to become part of every practice team's performance monitoring procedures and should be viewed as contributing to the practice's overall purpose or 'mission'. Seen in this context, the establishment of precise procedures suitable for any particular practice are a function of its practice management (Chapter 10). However, the guidelines shown in Box 8.2 may help a practice team to determine what its approach should be.

It is essential to specify the purpose of confidential enquiries in writing, so that there is no possibility of misunderstanding. There are two basic purposes:

Box 8.2: Guidelines for practice confidential enquiries

- Specify the purpose
- Establish confidentiality rules
- Designate responsibility
- Make arrangements for identifying critical events
- Collect the evidence
- Consider the results
- Make necessary changes

---

1 to seek to learn from the exercise and so secure improvement;
2 to apportion blame.

If the intention is to secure improvement, which is the only sensitive way of using the method, it must be made clear that the temptation in individual cases to apportion blame will not be allowed.

Establishing the ground rules for confidentiality is an equally important task. The general principles of confidentiality in audit should apply (as described in Chapter 11), but in addition the practice team may choose to retain the results of any confidential enquiry within the practice. Alternatively, a practice may choose to release anonymized data to the MAAG or others at its discretion. In some cases, the use of anonymized patient files should be considered within a practice, to protect either the patient or an individual health professional. This is probably more appropriate in larger practices where some of the practice team may not have been involved in the case, than in smaller practices where it is likely that everyone will know of the initial problem.

It is helpful to have one named person take responsibility for organizing and conducting confidential enquiries. That person should collect data on all incidents, and decide which are to be explored further. The value of assigning responsibility is that the individual concerned will gain experience in the method. The named person should also be accountable to the partnership or practice team. The person responsible may wish to consult about individual cases, especially if a health professional in another discipline within the practice team was involved.

The method of choosing and collecting cases should be one that all members of the practice team knows can operate. Incidents may be reported from a variety of sources, for example, a patient complaint, by a partner or member of staff, by a local hospital or the social services, or through the practice's routine performance monitoring. The most important question to ask when choosing cases is:

'By looking at this event in more detail, is it likely that we will learn anything that will help avoid future error or otherwise secure improvement?'

The key to a successful confidential enquiry lies in collecting the evidence. The relevant facts may be in the patient's records, documented in the appointment system or visiting books, or may be gained by interviewing the individuals concerned. The presentation of the case history and the findings will form the basis for subsequent discussion.

Ideally, the discussion should involve the whole practice team, so that everyone can learn. However, an incident involving technical clinical matters should be discussed by either the medical members of the practice or the medical and nursing staff together. It is essential that the individual who has carried out the enquiry should *not* chair the discussion, but should present the case, being prepared to clarify aspects of the history or findings as necessary.

It is important to record the conclusions, and particularly any proposals for change because they may have wider implications for the practice. Such proposals should be fed back through the practice manager to the partnership for further consideration as part of the normal management process.

In the course of several confidential enquiries, it may become clear that certain individuals have patterns of performance that are not satisfactory. If this should occur, it is important that the practice uses procedures separate from those of audit to manage the situation. The established machinery within the practice for investigating complaints about misconduct or poor performance should be used.

Use of tracers

In assessing the quality of care, it is impossible to examine in detail every aspect of the work of individual clinicians or practice teams. The use of 'tracer' conditions may help to overcome this problem. A tracer is a single clinical condition, either a symptom or a disease entity, which is chosen to explore aspects of performance, usually by external review. In assessing the process and outcomes of care, the tracer condition chosen may be held to be representative of quality in similar conditions which are not being assessed. In Case Study 7, hypertension was used as a tracer condition to demonstrate the standard of care of chronic illness in a practice.

To be effective, tracers should meet the criteria shown in Box 8.3.

As multi-practice audits become more commonplace, tracers will be used increasingly. The use of tracers requires skill and resources for data handling, analysis and feedback, and therefore such audits are likely to be

---

Box 8.3: 'Tracer' criteria

- The condition should be easy to define.
- The condition should be amenable to improvement by medical care.
- There should be a sound basis for discriminating between good and unsatisfactory care for the condition.
- The effects of non-medical factors on the condition should be adequately understood.
- The condition should yield enough patients for audit.

Source: Kessner et al., 1973[6]

---

implemented by MAAGs and FHSAs which have the potential for handling them.

Practice visiting

The third method of audit described in this chapter involves a visit made to a practice by local peers or external assessors. This approach was founded on the external assessment of teaching practices by visiting peers. It was initially developed by the RCGP, but is used today by the JCPTGP and regional postgraduate organizations for the selection of training practices. There is evidence to show that the recently appointed MAAGs are using methods equivalent to a practice visit as a means of helping to establish audit in general practices in their own areas.

Method

In some cases, peer inspections can be relatively informal, but for most cases the method is more formalized. One of the best known is the RCGP[7] *What Sort of Doctor?* method, in which four areas are considered to be indicative of performance: professional values, accessibility, clinical competence and the ability to communicate. Data illustrating these aspects of performance can be obtained from routine statistics kept by the practice, clinical records, videos of consultations and interviews with the health professionals concerned. In New Zealand, a patient's representative is included in the visiting team, and data are also sought from patients about satisfaction with care given.

A further description of method is beyond the scope of this book, because practice visiting is an external audit. However, practitioners who are members of MAAGs and others who may be interested in the visiting method will find that detailed information is available from the office of the regional adviser in general practice, the JCPTGP (which carries out regular organizational audits of regional postgraduate organizations for accreditation purposes) and the RCGP[8], which has detailed documentation on the data required of a practice in connection with the assessments made for fellowship of the college.

Summary

Audit method and data collection are interrelated. They are the heart of audit. In this and the preceding chapter, we have attempted to show the range of data already available in the average practice, and how simple methods of data collection can make more data available relatively easily. The most popular audit methods, especially practice activity analysis and the analysis of individual cases, are within the scope of any practice team and taken together they make a useful starting point.

9 How to do it: Analysing and Feeding Back Information

The data collection grid

WHATEVER the initial objectives, and the methods chosen, any audit will produce a considerable amount of data. Example 9.1 gives a hypothetical situation.

Example 9.1

An audit was carried out of people aged over 75 years in one practice who were taking antihypertensive therapy. The practice team identified 40 cases, from the practice computer, the repeat prescription system, or through the opportunistic recording of cases when seen by the doctor. The basic demographic data about the patients were recorded: age, sex, and so on. Recording the time and level of the last blood pressure reading was important, as was recording the types of treatment and iatrogenic problems. These data were collected by practice activity analysis and a series of interviews. Each of the 40 cases yielded 20 items of data which were set out on a data selection grid (*see* Fig. 9.1).

As a result there were 800 (40 × 20) boxes or cells to complete in the grid. Not all the items in these boxes required 'Yes' or 'No' answers. Some included a range of options, such as marital status — single, widowed or married (S, W or M) — or the type of drug therapy — labelled a, b or c — thereby substantially increasing the potential number of data items.

Example 9.1 illustrates several points.

1 A considerable quantity of data can be generated by audit even when only a small number of cases are being examined. This underlines the importance of starting small and planning the audit according to the skills and data-handling resources available. It also reinforces the point made in Chapter 7: a data item should be collected only if it is necessary.

2 Any attempt at analysis will be frustrated unless a suitable method of organizing the data has been devised at the planning stage. In general, and particularly for smaller audits, all the data should be entered into a grid drawn on paper (*see* Fig. 9.1). This gives an overview essential to understanding the nature and quality of the information that can be

	1	2	3	4	5	6	→ 20
	Age	Sex	Drug	Marital status	BP recorded		
Case 1	94	M	A	S	Y		
Case 2	90	M	B	W	Y		
Case 3	87	F	C	M	N		
↓ 40							

Figure 9.1 Data collection grid

derived from the data. In practices where there is appropriate computer software and expertise, computerized spreadsheets can be used; for larger data sets, a simple analysis package is essential.

3 The data collected should be 'clean'. Inconsistencies need to be identified, for example:

- cases in which the age lies outside the chosen age range;
- misrecordings of sex or marital status;
- unusual combinations of events either due to error or an unusual care pattern.

The analysis

The analysis must reflect the aims of the audit. If the purpose was to examine the drugs that seemed to cause side-effects in older people on antihypertensive therapy, that should be the priority of the analysis. One of the dangers of computerized analysis is the capacity to examine many items. The laws of probability ensure that the more data which are examined, the greater the likelihood will be of revealing interesting patterns. However, this will distract from the original aim of the audit, and analysis should always be focussed.

The first step in any analysis is to examine the frequency of occurrence of each item or event. Thus, using the Example 9.1, eight out of the 40 people may be widowed, and 15 out of 40 may be taking two or more drugs. Each of these numbers could be expressed as percentages, although percentages should not be used unless there are 50 cases or more in any data set.

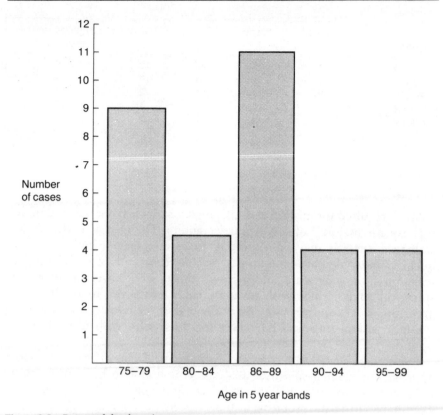

Figure 9.2 Range of database items

The next step is to construct a table that shows the range of each item of data collected (*see* Fig. 9.2). The point of this exercise is to highlight unusual occurrences; analysis can then be focussed on these events.

If some of the key data items or variables are not well represented within a range, for instance, there may be only one person in each annual age-group, grouping the cases together in a logical way that fits an agreed convention can overcome this problem. Ages can be grouped in 5-year bands: 75–79, 80–84, 85–89, and so on.

As a result, part of the analysis should be to produce one or more tables containing only the data required. For instance, the data in Fig. 9:1 can be summarized as shown in Fig. 9.3.

Statistical analysis

Summary statistics based on simple techniques, such as proportions or means together with frequencies or counts, form the basis for much of the

Age (years)	Married	Single	Total	BP recorded	Antihypertensive prescribed
75–79	9	3	12	13	0
80–84	4	2	6	10	1
85–89	3	7	10	2	1
90–94	2	6	8	1	0
95–99	1	3	4	2	
Total	9	21	40	28	2

Figure 9.3   Data presentation card

analysis required for medical audit. Complex statistical analysis is unnecessary for the majority of single practice audits. The idea of undertaking a statistical analysis may be offputting to certain team members. Consequently, this section has concentrated on simple methods of analysis and the techniques of generating information; those who have an interest in statistical analysis may wish to apply such techniques to results where appropriate. The short reading list at the end of the book contains some of the more useful statistical references for those who wish to explore this option.

Recent developments in computer software packages offer an alternative approach to manual statistical analysis. It is useful to have access to an analysis package that will facilitate comparisons. For instance, when examining iatrogenic problems in frail, elderly people receiving antihypertensive therapy, as in Example 9.1, it may be necessary to detect any differences between men and women at different ages.

Two groups of patients, male and female, would have to be selected and then tables constructed such as those shown in Fig. 9.4.

Comparisons could also be made with patients who are *not* taking the

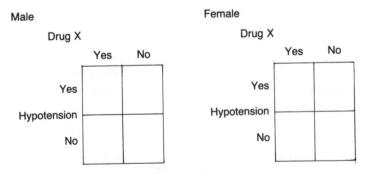

Figure 9.4   The tabulation that would show the distribution of hypotensive symptoms in males and females, receiving or not receiving drug X

drug in question, e.g. untreated controls. However, the volume of work involved if such comparisons have to be done manually (aided by a calculator) is large. Fortunately, the software now available can be run on a practice micro-computer; one such package is called EpiInfo, the details of which are included in the references to this chapter at the end of the book.[1]

Presentation of data

The analysis of data produces results that need to be converted into information which the practice team can understand and to which they can relate. Many health professionals are not used to interpreting data and are discouraged by tables that summarize many facts. Trends or insights must be presented in a visual way that communicates the information effectively.

To return to Example 9.1, suppose there are six different permutations of therapeutic regimen which the patients under study could be taking:

Thiazides only	4
Methyldopa	2
Beta-blockers	10
Ace inhibitors	4
Beta-blockers and thiazide	12
None	8
Not taking therapy	8

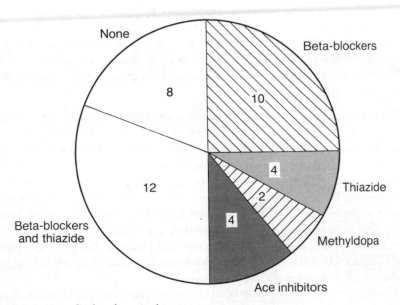

Figure 9.5   Data displayed as pie chart

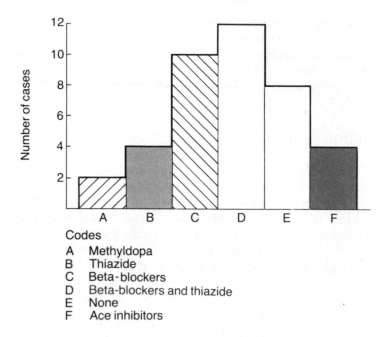

Codes
A   Methyldopa
B   Thiazide
C   Beta-blockers
D   Beta-blockers and thiazide
E   None
F   Ace inhibitors

Figure 9.6   Data displayed as bar chart

This information can be presented graphically by the use of a pie chart, as in Fig. 9.5, or a bar chart, as in Fig. 9.6. Simple graphics programmes can be run on personal computers; EpiInfo is easy to use in this respect. Alternatively, local schools or colleges are often willing to provide graphical skills.

There are sound reasons for spending time on ensuring the acceptability of the presentation of the data.

1 The information may be disturbing to some team members. No practice can provide consistently high quality in all aspects of health care. The purpose of audit is to highlight particular aspects of performance, and inevitably there will be times when elements of performance will fall below stated objectives. Whatever the mechanism the practice team has for feeding back audit results, it needs to take into account the potential for finding uncomfortable results and how those results are to be handled. The management framework within a practice necessary to ensure that such presentations lead to effective and planned changes is discussed in Chapter 10. Case Study 10 provides an illustration of what happens when such a framework does not exist.

2 Effective presentation assists accurate interpretation (*see* Chapter 7); in Case Study 15, an audit of the care of patients with diabetes shows how

presentation can help a practice to distinguish between an improvement in patient care resulting from better drug management and an improvement in the standard of record-keeping. If it had been presented in the form of tables, it may have been harder for colleagues to interpret the information correctly.

Summary

The purpose of feedback is to allow health professionals to compare the information obtained with their initial explicit standards, to debate the issues raised, to question performance and to make proposals for improvement where appropriate. Without effective practice management to ensure that such proposals are implemented and that changes are monitored (to confirm that improvement is attained and maintained), the process of audit is pointless. For this reason, in Chapter 10, the management context for the practice team and for the audit is discussed, and the importance of setting audit into a wider area is emphasized.

10 How to do it: Management and Managing Change

Audit and management

MANY papers and books on audit in general practice stop here, the audit chosen, the data collected, the results presented and perhaps changes identified. But then what? Too often a practice is content to leave it at that, comfortable in the knowledge that the results were interesting, the process was educational (and PGEA accredited), and there remains the good intention to make some changes in some unspecified way, at some unspecified time in the future.

This book began by saying that, in three fundamental respects, there is an explicit and direct connection between audit and the way a practice is managed:

1 in the definition of objectives and setting of standards;
2 in the monitoring and assessment of performance;
3 in the management of change.

The emphasis throughout has been on the integration of audit with practice management, and the value of audit in improving patient care, the quality of life for the health professionals involved, and, in many cases, the income of the practice. The reasons for devoting a chapter to the management framework are as follows.

1 The effective translation of the changes identified by audit into altered activities or priorities within the practice is a requirement, not an option.
2 In the same way that good management is vital to worthwhile audit, the regular auditing, or monitoring, of activities is an essential part of a practice's management plan. Specific audits, and the monitoring of overall performance against predetermined objectives, are integral to modern practice management.
3 The processes described in this book relating to the audit cycle (Fig. 3.1), particularly the definition of objectives and planning, and the need for reliable data and teamwork, are common to audit and management; one informs the other.

This chapter introduces the management cycle and sets audit in the wider context of the overall management needs of a practice. As planning is as important in the management cycle as it is in the audit cycle, the production of a written development plan for the practice is also discussed. The development plan is a sign of active planning in a practice, and it provides a suitable framework for prioritizing audit; a development plan is also dependent upon audit for effective construction.

The context: overall management needs

In general practice, the quality of care is dependent upon the attitudes, skills and knowledge of each individual working either separately or in concert with colleagues, and upon the deployment of these factors in the organization as a whole. Quality care is also the result of planned care, especially in the management of chronic diseases, preventive medicine, and acute illness. In order to provide planned care, practices require the policies, organization and management skills, information systems and appropriate arrangements necessary for audit. In turn, planned care requires teamwork, and sound data for effective decision-making, especially when determining the aims, objectives and priorities for care, and identifying the criteria and standards from which the performance of individuals and the practice team will be audited.

Management combines strategic and operational activities. The starting point for management is effective teamwork and communication.

Teamwork is the means whereby people work together to achieve a defined common goal. A team begins to develop when those involved have a shared purpose. When the members of a team integrate skills to accentuate strengths and minimize weaknesses, the practice objectives are usually achieved; groups that work as a collection of individuals usually fail.

The concept of teamwork was introduced to general practice 30 years ago when the movement towards group practice began, and nurses and health visitors were attached to practices in growing numbers. The reason for promoting teamwork is that much of primary care is shared, especially the management of patients who have a chronic illness, postoperative care following early discharge after surgery, and in preventive medicine. The feature that distinguishes teamwork in hospital from that in primary care is that in primary care each team member provides care for the patient alone and unsupervised in the consulting room, in the treatment room or in the patient's home. In a hospital team the members tend to work alongside one another on the same patient, for example, in the operating theatre.

Effective teamwork requires effective leadership. In the context of the clinical requirements of care in general practice, co-ordination is the challenge most partners have to meet, because they are cast in a traditional leadership role. Leadership qualities are required in order to achieve cooperation, and to manage disparate activities and individuals to a single endpoint. Leaders should be self-confident, optimistic, strong and considerate.

They have to be both powerful and popular, strong and yet persuasive. The successful implementation of any plan depends to a large extent on the quality of the original planning and the organization that preceded it, but also on sound leadership that gives support and encouragement to all members of staff.

It is widely acknowledged that the implementation of teamwork in general practice is patchy (Gregson et al., 1991)[1]. There may be three important reasons for this.

1 General practitioners, by the very nature of their jobs, have acquired attitudes and a professional ethos that favour independent action often at the expense of concerted effort. It is this ethos that stresses the value of personal rather than shared care.
2 As a consequence, practice members are not accustomed to defining common, i.e. team objectives, criteria and standards, even when they are looking after the same patients. This is because the value of an active planning process in primary care that would include performance review or audit has not been widely recognized.
3 There has been little monitoring of patients whose care is shared by all team members, because the means to do so has not existed.

However, a well-managed practice should ensure that all individuals work together as a team when appropriate. Mutual support and understanding of personal and team goals, and a climate of trust in which honest communicaton is encouraged, are vital to effective audit. The importance of presenting the results of audit in a non-threatening way was emphasized in Chapter 9. However well this may be done, the importance of creating a 'safe' environment in which the team can discuss potentially uncomfortable findings is vital. Effective teams include members who are encouraged to develop skills, apply what they learn and contribute to the success of the practice by using their individual talents and knowledge to achieve a common purpose.

What is management?

For many people especially general practitioners, the word 'management' conjures up visions of control, paperwork, bureaucracy, rules and discipline. However its purpose is to bring order out of chaos. Management is primarily about getting things done through people who come together within an organization to create objectives and then implement them. It is important to bear in mind that events and people do not always conform, plans need to be continually revised and amended to reflect changes. In management it is important to experiment with different approaches to old and new problems.

Many general practitioners dislike management because they view it only in terms of practice organization; in other words, management is confused with administration. The distinction, frequently blurred, can be clarified by understanding that management falls into three operations (Fig. 10.1).

1 The process of 'visioning' or of formulating the policies from which strategies are devised and the operational management has to implement. The 'vision' is the answer to the question 'Why is the practice here?'.

> **Policy:**   *Why* the organization is there
> **Strategy:**   *What* it intends to do to enact its policy
> **Operations:**   *How* it will implement the strategy
>
> Source: Huntingdon J (1991)[2]

Figure 10.1   The management function

2 Devising the strategies necessary to pursue the long-term aims or policies to relate the context in which a general practice team works to future aspirations and needs.
3 Operational (or administrative) management which is concerned with the running of a general practice, and the implementation of well-established systems within clear guidelines. It is initially about allocating resources. It embraces the problems of appraising priorities, assessing skill-mix, finding different ways of doing things and identifying new resources where appropriate.

The management cycle

The commonly recognized constituent activities of management are:

- planning;
- organizing;
- motivating;
- co-ordinating;
- monitoring.

These constituents can be more readily shown as a cycle (Fig. 10.2).

The final part of the cycle, i.e. monitoring, is the point where audit is directly relevant. The audit cycle shown in Fig. 3.1 can be seen as an enlargement of the monitoring part of the management cycle. Both cycles are continuous processes, as the auditing or monitoring of performance

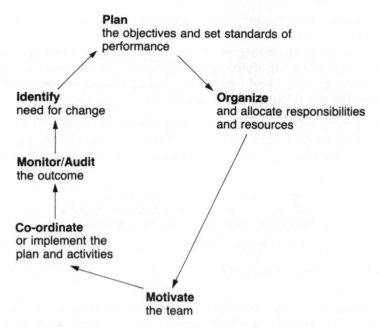

Figure 10.2 The management cycle

against planned objectives feeds into a review of the practice team's objectives and activities. As stated earlier, audit reveals the changes necessary which can illumine a practice's review of its plans, and which ought to be implemented, thereby forming part of the plans.

Why plan?

Planning is the starting point of the management cycle, as it is of the audit process. Planning is necessary because it gives a sense of direction, it focusses the resources of the practice on key objectives, and it provides answers to the following questions:

- Where are we now?
- Where do we want to be?
- How can we get there?
- How will we know when we have arrived?
- If we do not arrive will we know why?

This process of reviewing a practice and making its purposes explicit is fundamental; it is also important to share agendas. If the career expectations of individual members of the practice team differ, and these differences are not explained or monitored, conflict may result. Lack of agreement about the aims of a practice can cause resistance to change. In Case Study 14 audit was used to revive a demoralized and frustrated practice team; it provides an example of how the integration of audit results and management processes is essential to practice direction.

Today, general practitioners are subject to a changing culture in which it is likely that professional and financial rewards will be given to those who plan effectively. Planned care is pro-active and explicit; unplanned care is reactive, leaving much unstated, such that other professionals would find it difficult to understand the process of care in a practice and its objectives.

The choice between planned and unplanned care may have practical consequences. For example, obtaining substantial financial backing from banks could be difficult without evidence of coherent planning, especially in written form. Similarly, seeking support from FHSAs or DHAs for expanding services (or the maintenance of existing services) is unlikely to be successful in the future without a clear indication from the practice team of what is to be achieved and how.

Benefits of development planning

It is becoming increasingly common for the planning stage of a management cycle to be written down. A 'development plan' is the description of a practice's current situation, the team's aspirations, and the means of getting from here to there, and assessing whether it has arrived[3,4]. The possible headings and structure for a conventional development plan are shown in Fig. 10.3 which is not intended as a blueprint, merely an example. Making the plan explicit clarifies the issues facing a practice team and enables it to identify workable solutions. The thought and discussion involved in generating a business plan are as important as the outcome. Writing down a development plan is a visible sign of the planning process. It can provide a secure framework within which the practice's audit activities can be planned and prioritized.

However, the benefits of a business plan need to be tangible to ensure commitment. Such benefits are listed in Box 10.1.

How to plan

In devising and drafting a development plan all team members should be involved, particularly those party to the management of the practice. It is essential that a practice devotes 'protected' time to this process. Time is

1 **Overall purpose**		What are we now and where are we going, broadly and more specifically?
'Mission' and aims		
Activities		What do we have to do to get there?

2 **Resources**		
Time	Data	What do we need to get there?
Money	Organizations	
People	Systems	
Capital stock	Protocols	

3 **Constraints/Strengths**	
Identify constraints	
Internal and external to the practice	What are the current constraints and what are we likely to meet in the future?
Identify strengths	
Internal and external to the practice	What factors are working in our favour now and what are likely to arise in the future?

4 **Monitoring of performance**	
The standard setting/performance review cycle	How will we know when and if we have got there?
	If we don't make it, will we know why?

Source: Irvine D (1990)[3]

Figure 10.3   The development plan

necessary for effective brainstorming; ideas should not be constrained by resource considerations, or political necessity.

Different groupings of team members can generate different perspectives of practice aims; for example, nurses, receptionists or partners can meet separately to brainstorm about the practice. When each group has finalized their ideas, all groups should meet to discuss them. An external facilitator can often help team members to overcome the traditional relationships and modes of expression within a practice. Although the process can be time-consuming, a general practice team with a common purpose or 'mission' is strong.

As the business plan will be the result of team effort, the process requires delegation to specific groups and individuals.

Box 10.1: The benefits of development planning

A development plan:

- ensures that the actions of the practice are fitted to its strategic direction;
- can help build a feeling of corporateness, without discouraging personal innovation.
- identifies explicitly the choices and the changes that have to be made;
- focusses on balancing the aspirations of the practice, in terms of the services it wishes to provide, against the resources available, in terms of money, staff, estate and equipment;
- identifies which factors are critical to success;
- requires the practice to assess explicitly the risk factors involved in its plans;
- identifies the different consumers of the practice's services (including the staff) and allows more effective and targeted marketing.

Delegation

Delegation is an arrangement whereby certain team members take on particular tasks or roles within a practice. Delegation can reveal a hidden core of resources and can be used to put existing skills to better effect. The appropriate delegation of administrative tasks can release other team members to perform the strategic tasks for which they have the expertise, and are able to take responsibility. Delegation can also increase personal development, resulting in greater job satisfaction and the enhancement of an individual's skills. For example, a receptionist given total responsibility for some activities may perform them more effectively than a relatively mindless task. Delegation confers ownership; ownership often leads to innovation and pride in a job well done.

There is no easy way to learn to delegate. In general it is important to ensure that the task being delegated is clearly defined and that appropriate support and authority are given to the delegatee. It is also important to ensure that the delegator understands the need to let go, to accept mistakes or praise success. Most importantly, supervision and monitoring appropriate to the task should be given. Finally, it is important that both the delegator and the delegatee feel confident about tasks delegated. The rules of good delegation are set out in Box 10.2.

Box 10.2: The rules of delegation

- Never do the work that others can do
- Think carefully about why you are delegating a task
- Set out the process of control and review
- Delegate the entire job
- Delegate adequate resources
- Ensure complete understanding in the delegatee
- Criticize the delegatee in private
- Ask others what you can delegate to them
- Retain responsibility for the results
- Use delegation to criticize your own performance

Source: Irvine S, 1987[5]

Motivation

Effective management and effective delegation are very dependent on an understanding of what motivates colleagues. The priority that work assumes for any individual is determined by many personal factors including background, age, status, family, involvement in other responsibilities, or in sporting, artistic or other endeavours. People have many reasons for working: to express their particular brand of creativity: to contribute to the social good; to earn a living; to earn enough to finance some valued leisure activities; to enjoy the social relationship work offers; to give some structure to the day and some purpose to life. They also have many reasons for working in a particular job. Motivation is essential to ensure the effective implementation of any management decision, and in this case the decision to perform an audit and implement any change arising.

There is a tendency to attach more importance to the technical roles of staff than to their motivational needs. An understanding of an individual's role within the wider context of the practice will generate commitment, which is particularly important when policies have to be implemented that involve change. Good communication will motivate people to understand the reasons for any changes that affect them. It is not sufficient to expect loyalty to be a prime motivator. Indeed, the greater the skills and professionalism of an individual, the more sophisticated the motivating factors are likely to be. Those factors usually identified as being the principal motivating forces for most people are listed in Box 10.3.

Box 10.3: Motivational factors

- A sense of ownership of a task or piece of work.
- The opportunity to plan and execute that work with a reasonable degree of freedom.
- The opportunity to test and prove one's capacity and judgement.
- Unobtrusive support from a manager.
- Feedback on the products and the process of the work (i.e. what has been achieved and the way it has been achieved).
- Recognition of achievement and growth (not necessarily in financial terms), i.e. being given more responsibility or greater status.

Managing change

Nowadays, the management of change has become an end in itself, and yet it is only one component of good management. Good managers are rarely taken by surprise; they plan ahead, they scan the horizon, they look for all possible pitfalls, and decide upon alternative strategies and tactics. If change is required, a good manager has the ability to handle it. Crisis management is a short-term solution which can be extremely draining on the personnel involved, particularly in general practice where team members are already subject to considerable stress.

A crisis is a change that an organization has not planned to meet. Therefore one of the major purposes of planning is to anticipate change. The anticipation of change is made easier if the need for change can be identified; a function of audit is to identify the need for change.

There is no quick and easy way of managing change. But all the issues that create tension and resistance — uncertainty about competence, fear of reducing status, or innovation being taken as a criticism of what went before — all perceptions of 'threat' can be turned on their hands into levers for beneficial change or opportunities.

Several factors are central to managing change — *see* Fig. 10.4 for a pictorial guide. In summary, it is essential to communicate the need for, and the impact of, change, to those likely to be involved at an early stage. If it is a change resulting from audit, appropriate planning of an audit will have ensured that the team members likely to be affected will have been involved in collecting the data and interpreting the results.

In any organization, it is important to recognize that change is not only necessary but normal: the only certainty is uncertainty. It is also important to present innovation or change as a benefit for patients. This can help to

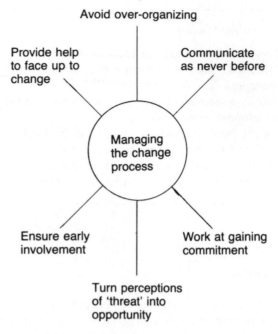

Source: Plant (1987)[6]

Figure 10.4   Managing change

engage commitment to the proposed change as can ensuring appropriate rewards. Planning is the most significant factor in ensuring a pro-active and managed approach to change.

Conclusion

The management of a general practice requires the same techniques and skills as the management of any business. These techniques involve being able to make the right choice between competing demands, and deciding on the most appropriate use of resources. Good management also includes knowing how to delegate, how to communicate effectively, how to plan, how to set objectives and how to monitor achievement. They cover knowing how to lead and how to support, how to encourage and motivate, how to cooperate, how to take responsibility, how to take decisions and how to exercise authority.

The effective management of a practice is vital to improve the standards of patient care and to ensure that these standards have been achieved. Without effective audit, this is not possible, and without the management framework within which audit can function and its results be implemented, audit is worthless.

11 Confidentiality

No guidance or audit would be complete without a consideration of the question of confidentiality within audit, in relation to both patients and health professionals.

Confidentiality and the patient

In any practice, audit should be conducted within the framework of confidentiality that already regulates clinical care. General Medical Council (GMC) guidelines[1] state that confidentiality should be preserved, except when the release of information may be specifically permitted, provided that the doctors can justify their action. There are similar guidelines from the United Kingdom Council for Nursing, Midwifery and Health Visiting (UKCC)[2] governing the relationship of nurses with their patients. Clinical confidentiality may extend beyond the individual doctor to other practitioners and members of the practice team concerned with the care of a patient. In general, it is accepted by the GMC and by lay organizations, in this country and abroad, that it is in the best interests of patients that health professionals within a practice should have access to medical records in confidence for the purpose of improving standards of patient care, i.e. for *internal* audit.

However, audit is not always internal; it may involve access to patient records by visiting peers, as in visits to training practices. The GMC has given guidance on training practice visiting which is relevant and can be applied to all practice audit activity. In its annual report in 1986[3], the GMC recommended that the existing arrangements for training practice inspections should continue, but specified that all doctors carrying out such inspections should act with sensitivity and discretion, and be conscious that they are bound by professional secrecy. The GMC also recommended that each training practice should ensure that all of its patients were informed of the circumstances in which their medical records might be disclosed to other doctors, for educational purposes. Such information can be given to patients via practice leaflets and notices in the surgeries. The GMC concluded with a statement that all patients have the right to refuse access to their medical records for audit purposes.

Confidentiality and doctors

During the operation of medical audit, doctors will be concerned that their names are protected. This concern is acknowledged in the DoH health circulars on audit[4,5]. This aspect of audit and confidentiality can be considered at two levels: within the practice, and in the relationship between the practice and the outside world.

It is important that a practice establishes policy guidance on confidentiality and internal audit because internal audit could reveal aspects of individual performance that previously had not been obvious or thought important. There are two ways of managing this situation.

1 The practice can decide that all matters revealed by an internal audit should remain private, especially if the performance of individual health professionals is concerned. The practice should also decide what to publish, and the form of publication.
2 The practice should consider an internal policy on anonymization. This is likely to apply to the confidential enquiry audit (Chapter 8, page 59) in which a particular health professional's name may not be relevant to the purpose and conduct of the audit. The easiest way to handle this aspect in practice is to apply the 'need to know' principle on each individual occasion.

In terms of the relationship between the practice and the outside world, it is important to determine MAAG policies on confidentiality, and to ensure that the practice policy complies. In general, MAAGs and any other external auditing bodies are advised to use anonymized data wherever possible. In the early stages of implementing audit, it is difficult to envisage situations where such data will not suffice. GMSC and RCGP policy is that nothing should be sent from a practice to a MAAG which would identify either the general practitioner or the patient. Legal advice has confirmed that information held by MAAGs could be subpoenaed by the courts.

It cannot be emphasized too strongly that, particularly at the level of the practice, privacy is of the utmost importance if honesty and trust are to be combined in the pursuit of improvement.

Confidentiality and professional obligations

One of the commonest questions asked about the operation of audit is: 'What should happen if less than satisfactory performance is revealed?' This sharpens even more the question of privacy and anonymity. The GMC has recently issued guidance to doctors to cover the situation when a practitioner has to comment on a colleague's professional practice. Although this situation can arise in several circumstances, it is likely to be of particular relevance in audit procedures. It is worthwhile noting in full the GMC's guidance to doctors[1] in such circumstances.

> 'Honest comment is entirely acceptable ... provided that it is carefully considered and can be justified, that it is offered in good faith and that it is intended to promote the best interests of patients.
>
> Further, it is any doctor's duty, where the circumstances so warrant, to inform an appropriate person or body about a colleague whose professional conduct or fitness to practice may be called in question, or whose professional performance appears to be in some way deficient. Arrangements exist to deal with such problems, and they must be used in order to ensure that high standards of medical practice are maintained.
>
> However, gratuitous and unsustainable comment which, whether directly or by implication, sets out to undermine trust in a professional colleague's knowledge or skills is unethical.'

This is the guidance which practices undertaking audit should follow.

12 Audit — Looking Ahead

IN this chapter the history of audit is outlined, and the setting of audit in the context of the MAAGs is explored. Knowledge of the history gives greater understanding of the subject, and the role of MAAGs may ensure a sense of direction.

Historical outline

One of the themes of this book is that the best way to learn about audit is to do it; it is also vital to relate practical experience to the theory and method of the subject through complementary reading and discussion. Much of the theory and method of medical audit originated in the USA; even today, much of the literature is North American. It is important to acknowledge the work of our American colleagues in developing this aspect of medical practice as well as to emphasize the significance of their literature in medicine worldwide. The World Health Organization has done much to show the relevance of audit's theoretical framework to medicine in any country, thereby dispelling the idea that audit has little relevance to European or British general practice.

The literature on audit in general practice is not extensive. In the UK, the starting point was studies in the 1950s and 1960s, which described the nature of general practice (Hadfield, 1953[1]; Taylor, 1954[2]), and also those that concentrated on describing the structural characteristics of general practice, i.e. the quality of the buildings, equipment, staffing and organization of general practice (Collings, 1950[3]; Irvine and Jeffreys, 1971[4]). The classic studies from North America (Petersen, et al., 1956[5]), Canada (Clute, 1963[6]) and Australia (Jungfer and Last, 1964[7]) at that time concentrated on the process of care, i.e. the complex of interactions between doctors and their patients.

In the 1970s and 1980s, increasing numbers of individual British general practitioners and practices performed and reported the results of practice audit (for example Barly and Mathers, 1980[8]; Colmer and Gray, 1983[9]; Hart, 1975[10]; Marsh, 1977[11]). These individual assessments were mainly about the process of care, and therefore the results described such activities as prescribing patterns, hospital referral patterns and the functioning of appointment systems or recall arrangements for screening programmes. Those planning an audit for the first time will find it helpful to read through some of the earlier work; the ideas, and the reports on the results of clinical care, are valuable because they are based on experience.

It is likely that the literature from British general practice will grow as more practices or groups of practices decide to publish their results (*see* latest literature review[12]). The plethora of reports, review articles and books on audit, which are becoming available mean that all those involved in primary health care delivery have ready access to material from which to learn about audit and to plan their own practice audits.

The future

The MAAG

Established general practitioners should be aware of the new elements of audit that have been introduced by the National Health Service, most notably the MAAGs, when considering their strategy in practice audit activity.

MAAGs are committees of the FHSAs, and their principal responsibilities are shown in Box 12.1.

Box 12.1: The principal responsibilities of MAAGs

Each MAAG will be accountable to the FHSA for:

- the institution of regular and systematic medical audit in which all practitioners take part, perhaps facilitated by the existence of local groups. The objective is the participation of all practices by April 1992;
- adequate procedures that ensure reports are cast in such a form that individual patients and doctors cannot be identified;
- establishing appropriate mechanisms to ensure that problems revealed through audit are solved and that the profession plays a full part in this;
- providing the FHSA with a regular report on the general results of the audit programme.

Source: DoH (1990)[13]

The MAAGs are to be led by the medical profession, and expected to build on the foundation of the existing commitment of general practitioners to the principles of self-audit and performance review. In this regard, they will have a strong educational element.

The MAAGs appear to be conscious of the need to develop a suitable guiding philosophy, and thereby inspire confidence within the medical profession. Many MAAGs are adopting an attitude of encouragement, and have offered support to practices in the form of audit facilitators, advice and further education and training.

All MAAGs are expected to have at least one adviser who has a sound working knowledge of the principles and methods of medical audit in general practice. These advisers are expected to facilitate the work of the MAAGs by providing the information and understanding necessary for making decisions in which everyone will have confidence. The importance of choosing an appropriate chairman has also been emphasized. Ideally, the person chosen should have leadership qualities that are obvious to the profession locally and to the FHSA, and he/she should be prepared to acquire a good working knowledge of the principles of audit. It is clear that the MAAG should become the local information point to which practice teams in the FHSA can turn for help and advice, particularly on the local facilities available.

The MAAGs have a representative of the teaching organizations within general practice among their members; the importance of the link between education and audit has been emphasized. In this connection, the MAAG and the office of the regional adviser in general practice will co-operate to identify the educational needs of practitioners and other members of the practice team, and to provide courses, and other educational activities, locally to meet these needs.

These educational activities are likely to encompass courses in basic audit methodology, including the construction of criteria and standards, and the wherewithal of how to do audit as outlined in this book.

By April 1992, the MAAG will have an established role in general practice within the NHS. Becoming familiar with the local MAAG, who the people are and how it is proposing to work will be something that every practice will want to do, perhaps most easily through the role of the partner who has responsibility for medical audit within a practice, or that of the practice manager.

Inevitably MAAGs are attracting a lot of attention and interest because they are new and intended by NHS management to promote quality in primary health care. It would be very easy for MAAGs to become the driving force for audit with individual practices adopting a reactive attitude, content simply to carry out policies and projects devised for them. This situation will not arise if individual practices take the lead because they have the motivation, knowledge and skill to manage quality themselves.

In the final analysis patients and health professionals will be best served by practices which themselves ensure quality within an enabling framework provided by the FHSA and its MAAG.

Suggested reading

References for specific chapters and case studies are set out at the end of the book, and provide a reading list in themselves.

The following is offered as those most likely to complement and extend the thoughts of this book.

Abrahamson H J (1987) *Survey methods in community medicine.* Churchill Livingstone, London.

Coulter A, Roland M, Wilkin D (1991) *GP referrals to hospital: a guide for family health services authorities.* Centre for Primary Care Research, Manchester.

Baker R & Presley P (1990) *The practice audit plan: a handbook of medical audit.* Royal College of General Practitioners, Severn Faculty.

Handy C (1989) *The age of unreason.* Business Books, London.

Hughes J & Humphreys C (1990) *Medical audit in general practice: a practical guide.* King Edward's Hospital Fund for London, London.

Hunt J (1986) *Managing people at work.* McGraw-Hill, London.

Irvine D H (1990) *Managing for quality in general practice.* King Edward's Hospital Fund for London, London.

Marinker M (ed.) (1990) *Medical audit in general practice.* British Medical Journal, London.

McIver S (1991) *Obtaining the views of users of health services.* King Edward's Hospital Fund for London, London.

Royal College of General Practitioners (1986) *Management in practice.* Video and coursebook. MSD Foundation for RCGP, London.

Royal College of General Practitioners (1990) *Who Killed Susan Thompson?* Video and coursebook. MSD Foundation for RCGP, London.

Section II

THE second half of this book is devoted to descriptions of audits that have been collected by the contributors from their own and neighbouring practices. They are previously unpublished, and not the result of research work. They are varied in complexity, rigour and success. They have been presented in a common format for ease of reference, but their strength lies in the reality of the situations they describe.

They provide a series of illustrations of the points made in Section I. They can be used as models or inspirations. They are set out in an order approximating to the list of benefits of audit as detailed in Chapter 2. However, one audit may illustrate more than one benefit. The audits described also use a variety of the data sources and methods, which are described in Chapters 7 and 8.

Readers can read the case studies without reference to the text, or may prefer to refer to them as encountered as cross references in Section I. For instance, Case Study 11 is an example of a confidential enquiry audit and it may be helpful to read it together with the section on confidential enquiries in Chapter 8; when reading Case Study 10, which illustrates practice activity analysis, it may be useful to read the section in Chapter 7 to expand upon the contents of the case study. References to relevant texts are given as appropriate, although the editors have resisted introducing too many in the interests of readability.

14 List of Case Studies

No.	Subject	Method
1	Reviewing the effectiveness of a Well Man Clinic, and the consequent use of resources.	Practice activity using informal contact data
2	Reviewing the effectiveness of a screening programme for a practice's 'over 75s'.	Proforma
3	Reviewing the impact of a screening service with a practice standard for epilepsy care.	Self-administered patient questionnaire
4	Reducing clinical error by comparing performance with a practice standard for epilepsy care.	Records review
5	Improving the effectiveness of rubella immunization amongst adolescent girls.	Practice activity analysis
6	Reducing clinical error in the use of H_2-antagonists.	Case review
7	Demonstrating the standard of care in hypertension.	Tracer condition
8	Reviewing organizational error.	Organization review
9	Identifying whether opportunistic screening is most effective method of ensuring that patients between 20 and 80 years have blood pressure checked.	Computer review of patient lists
10	Identifying reasons for frustration and irritation.	1 Practice activity analysis 2 Patient satisfaction 3 Confidential enquiry
11	Reducing clinical and organizational error.	Confidential enquiry

12	Assessing effectiveness of changed approach to delivery of diabetes care.	Records review
13	Assessing patterns of referral practice.	Practice activity analysis using data collecting sheet
14	Improving effectiveness and efficiency of rubella immunization.	Audit of process/ intermediate outcome using routine practice data
15	Improving glycaemic control in diabetic patients.	Disease index and patient records

Case Study 1

Subject of audit

A process audit reviewing the efficiency and effectiveness of a 'well man' clinic and the consequent use of resources, using practice activity analysis and routine practice data.

Background

A nurse-led 'well man' clinic had been established in the practice, to offer health checks to men aged 30–60 years as part of the health promotion programme. The practice nurse had been given a major role in its planning and institution, protocol development and in implementation. A postal call and recall system was used to contact the selected population of men aged 30–60 years. A standard letter was produced which provided an appointment time, the aims of the clinic and a brief description of what would happen. Appointments were booked such that the clinic was in operation for one day of the week. A three-year cycle was planned for these health checks.

The administrative tasks were the responsibility of one of the reception staff. These tasks included the identification of patients from the age–sex register, making appointments, sending out letters and recording the attenders and non-attenders.

Reason for the audit

As one of the partners remarked,

'It would be nice to say that this audit was part of a general policy of looking at what we were doing. Regrettably most of us only look at our work when a problem is identified and this audit was no different!'

The doctors and nurses felt that the turnout at the clinic was low, particularly for younger men. Too much nurse time seemed to be lost in waiting for patients who were booked but did not turn up. The nurse also wondered if she was providing a valuable service — did she really pick up any significant illnesses or concerns amongst attenders?

Aims of audit

The audit was performed to test the impression that, in terms of turnout and positive findings by age, the clinic could be made more effective.

Methods

Routine practice activity data, entered into the appointment book and onto a specially designed proforma kept within the clinical record, were abstracted and analysed. In addition, when non-attenders at the clinics came to the surgery for another reason, they were asked why they had not attended the clinic, and their answers were collated.

Who carried out the audit?

One option was for a partner to conduct this audit. However, the task was given to the practice manager to delegate appropriately. The counting and initial analysis was carried out by the receptionist who had special responsibility for the clinic, and the further analysis by the practice manager, practice nurse and partners.

Results

The audit confirmed that turnout was very poor in the younger age-group, but improved with the increasing age of attenders (Table CS1.1).

Informal questioning by both doctors and nurses during other contact revealed the reasons for non-attendance. The clinic was held during working hours and, as most men saw no need for a health check because they felt

Table CS1.1 Turnout by age

Age (years)	Attenders (%)
30–39	37
40–49	45
50–59	55

Table CS1.2 Examples of frequency of positive findings by age

	Age (years)		
Findings	30–39	40–49	50–59
Urine abnormal	1.5%	3%	6%
PEF abnormal	22%	6%	34%
Blood pressure borderline (single reading)	22%	7%	32%
Blood pressure raised	0%	0%	6%
Non-smokers	62%	43%	33%
Non-drinkers	6%	9%	22%
Normal BMI	70%	94%	98%
Smokers at least 15 cigarettes/day	19%	18%	28%
Drinkers at least 30 units/week	20%	17%	12%

well, they did not attend. However, many became interested when it was discussed with them, and arranged an appointment.

The positive findings were difficult to interpret (Table CS1.2). 'Hard' factors, such as urine screening, had a minimal positive pick-up: < 5% overall showed any abnormality. Several men were found to have borderline hypertension which required further checking. The majority of the men who had had their level of serum cholesterol measured were found to have a level above the norm, consequent with national research findings. 'Soft' data, relating to smoking, alcohol and body mass index, were obtained which formed the basis for further health education.

The analysis showed defects in the organization of the clinic in that its timing was inconvenient, its purpose was not understood and it was not well advertised. The findings also demonstrated that further health education would be valuable in men with risk factors, such as smoking habit and excessive alcohol consumption.

Changes resulting from audit

It was obvious that major organizational changes were required.

1 The routine call and recall system was abandoned.
2 The clinic was advertised in the surgery.
3 Women attending for cervical cytology were informed of the service available for their partners.
4 Appointments were offered opportunistically when men attended for routine consultations. Thus, the overall allocation of appointments to a

specific day was changed to a more flexible arrangement guided by the convenience of the patient and nurse.

The problem of getting young men interested in health education formed the basis of a practice educational meeting; the practice nurse has undertaken further educational courses in smoking cessation; and specific protocols such as those for obesity management have been developed.

Was the audit repeated?

It was important to see if these developments produced any changes. The audit was repeated and revealed a far greater turnout of patients for these checks: over 90% of those who made appointments kept them. Consequently, the nurse was able to use her time more effectively. Although the pick-up of positive findings revealed much the same outcomes, the nurse's confidence in dealing with men with risk factors (smoking, drinking and obesity) had increased. Subsequent audits should reveal whether changes in patient behaviour lead to fewer smokers, reduced alcohol consumption, etc.

Comment

This audit is an example of a simple practice activity analysis (*see* Chapter 7) and helps to answer the question of efficiency. It is ideal for monitoring the activity produced by a well man clinic.

This audit suffered initially from poorly defined aims and objectives (*see* Chapter 5) which in turn reflected the inadequate planning of the clinic itself. In the future clinical protocols should be designed (*see* Chapter 6) and records which are 'audit-friendly' used. This will make regular performance monitoring easier.

Case Study 2

Subject of audit

A process audit reviewing the efficiency of a screening programme for the 'over 75' population against the programme's objectives, using a proforma to collect data.

Background

Several years ago, a practice decided to screen its elderly. The practice team met several times to review the available literature, after which it was agreed that the programme should assess primarily how the elderly functioned in their homes, rather than attempt to discover occult disease.

A standard proforma was used as a checklist for screening and also to facilitate the manual extraction of data at a later date. The 'at risk' population was identified using the practice's age–sex register. It was divided into those patients who regularly attended the surgery, those who had regular home visits, either from a doctor, district nurse or health visitor, and those with whom the practice had had no recent contact.

Opportunistic screening was performed by the member of the practice team who made the next suitable contact. Patients who rarely attended were sent a standard letter outlining the purpose of the programme and were made an offer of an appointment at the surgery or a home visit.

Reason for audit

As opportunistic screening is time-consuming, it was important that an assessment of the benefits to the elderly in relation to the effort involved should be made.

Aims of audit

The audit was designed to:

- measure the uptake of the service by the target population;
- assess/quantify the functional needs/deficits identified;

- find out whether non-attenders had important unfulfilled needs;
- assess the adequacy of the proforma.

Methods

The proforma was the primary data source. As the practice did not have a computer at that time, the proforma was structured in a form suitable for manual extraction by lay staff. A simple 'Yes/No response' format was used whenever possible, for example:

> Hearing problem present   Yes/No
> Hearing aid possessed   Yes/No
> If Yes, hearing aid used
> etc.

Who carried out the audit?

The data extraction and the subsequent analysis were carried out by one of the partners who was particularly enthusiastic about the project, and the practice manager. However, the exercise could have been performed equally well by the practice administrative staff under the guidance of the practice manager, which would have been more cost-effective.

Results

As other surveys of this age-group have shown, a variety of daily functional needs were revealed. Patients were identified who would benefit from hearing aids, spectacles, bath aids, meals on wheels, and so on. Data about dependency on others for help and recent bereavement were also obtained. A sample of some of the results is given in Table CS2.1.

The audit confirmed that the majority of people who make no demand on primary care, i.e. the group which did not seek medical advice regularly, had no major unmet needs. However, all the elderly questioned were positive in their attitude to the new service, and were impressed that their needs were being considered.

Table CS2.1   Elderly screening

Functional needs	%
Living alone	53
Depending on someone for help	56
Confined to home by ill health	36
Loss of someone close in last year	15
Concerned about current health	59
Recent visual problems	36
Recent hearing difficulties	27
Problems with bladder control	26

Changes resulting from audit

The resulting changes may be summarized as follows:

- as opportunistic screening gave the best yield, routine visits to people who were well were discontinued;
- the proforma was improved;
- an information sheet for patients was introduced;
- subsequent reviews of results were to be carried out every three years;
- the practice manager and her staff were to organize and carry out subsequent reviews, as part of the regular monitoring of a service to patients;
- there would be a further exploration of patient attitudes to practice services (*see* Case Study 3).

As the New Contract for general practice was introduced two years later, the programme had to be modified to comply. However, the changes were relatively easy to make, and are now being monitored, because the practice had already implemented the basic systems.

Benefits of audit to the practice

- The practice team established what they were doing.
- The basis for subsequent improvement could be readily identified, and so the desirable changes were easy to institute.
- Patient satisfaction with the services was documented.
- The practice team felt reassured that they were developing a service of benefit and value to patients, and which was becoming cost-effective.

Comment

This is another simple practice activity analysis (*see* Chapter 7) which was well planned and with testable aims. It was seen as an integral part of managing this part of the practice's services.

Case Study 3

Subject of audit

AN audit of process and outcome, reviewing the impact of a screening service for the elderly on patient satisfaction, using a self-administered patient questionnaire, and assessing whether this and similar services would improve the practice image.

Background

A recent audit (Case Study 2) by a practice team of the screening of its 'over 75' population had confirmed that, although most people who make no call on the practice services have no need of them, the elderly population were very positive about screening.

Reason for audit

A desire to find out more about the attitude of patients to planned preventive care offered by the practice, and to assess its effect on the practice image.

Aim of audit

To test the belief of the practice team that planned preventive services are welcomed by patients.

Method

The practice carried out a postal audit of patient satisfaction using a self-administered questionnaire with Likert scales. A representative sample of patients was drawn using the practice age–sex register. Results were collated and analysed by one partner and the practice manager.

An extract from the questionnaire is shown below.

'The practice is developing new preventive services for patients. Our aim is to stop illness before it starts and so hopefully ensure healthier and happier patients. Could you spend a few minutes answering some questions?

1. Did you know about the following services provided at the surgery?

Well Women checks	Yes	No	Unsure
Well Man checks	Yes	No	Unsure
Elderly checks	Yes	No	Unsure
. . . etc			

2. Which of the following services have you used?

Well Women checks	Yes	No	Unsure
Well Man checks	Yes	No	Unsure
Elderly checks	Yes	No	Unsure
. . . etc			

3. If you have not used these services would you be likely to in the future?

Well Women checks	Yes	No	Unsure
Well Man checks	Yes	No	Unsure
Elderly checks	Yes	No	Unsure
. . . etc			

4. Are there services we do not provide that you feel we should? Please comment if you wish.

5. In general I think the practive provides a good service.

1	2	3	4	5
strongly agree	agree	unsure	disagree	strongly disagree

6. The new preventive services are an improvement in the services of the practice.

1	2	3	4	5
strongly agree	agree	unsure	disagree	strongly disagree

7. The surgery hours are convenient to me.

1	2	3	4	5
strongly agree	agree	unsure	disagree	strongly disagree

Please comment if you wish.

8. I feel I could see a doctor today without an appointment if I felt I needed to.

1	2	3	4	5
strongly agree	agree	unsure	disagree	strongly disagree

and so on ...'

Results

The response rate varied by age. The elderly had the highest response rate of about 90%. Men between the ages of 30 and 65 years had the lowest response rate, that of 65%.

The survey provided useful information about patients' views on the practice's services. In terms of preventive care, the results suggested that overall patients preferred targeted preventive clinics to opportunistic screening. Conversely, patients who made little use of the practice currently indicated that they would be unlikely to make use of planned preventive services in future; however, they tended to believe that the services offered were 'a good thing' and improved their view of the practice.

Changes resulting from the audit

The results of the audit helped to:

• shape new preventive services;
• led to improvements in the practice leaflet;
• prompted the practice to explore further how it might gather patient's opinions and suggestions for improvement on a regular basis.

Was the audit repeated?

The next audit will focus on patient uptake and use of regular services for the acutely and chronically ill.

Comment

The practice had decided to carry out this particular audit because the results of the first audit (Case Study 2) had suggested that the practice image was improved by the provision of a particular service. The practice team decided to verify this impression because it could have important consequences for practice policy.

In the past, it was rare for doctors to carry out patient satisfaction surveys. It is important that such questionnaires are worded carefully to ensure that patients record what they really feel. In this particular case, the questionnaire was sent to a representative sample of patients, but it could have given very useful informaton had it been administered to surgery attenders at the conclusion of a consultation.

Patient satisfaction is one of the parameters that FHSAs have to measure under the New Contract. Although it is likely that such surveys will be performed at district level, it is important for practices to assess patient satisfaction within their individual populations. Audits of patient satisfaction should help a practice team to ensure that its services are what patients want, and that they are of an acceptable standard. They can be used as a tool to improve the practice image by showing that doctors care about their patients, and that they are prepared to respond to unmet needs.

Case Study 4

Subject of audit

A process audit attempting to reduce clinical error by comparing performance with a practice standard for the care of patients with epilepsy, using a records review.

Background

One of the advantages of having a trainee within a practice is that they can stimulate change. This particular practice had two trainees who had carried out an audit of the care of the patients with epilepsy in the practice in 1979. The outstanding finding for that audit was that over 50% of patients with epilepsy had not been seen by a doctor or nurse in the previous year.

As a result of the 1979 audit, the practice team formulated an explicit standard that every patient with epilepsy on medication should be reviewed at least once a year. As a consequence of this the practice team felt that a review of patients with epilepsy should show an improvement in patient contacts upon that revealed in 1979.

Reason for audit

Despite having a basic standard, the practice's handling of patients with epilepsy still seemed to be variable.

Aim of audit

To assess the degree of compliance with the practice criteria and standards.

Method

At the time of the audit, the practice had a manual diagnostic index including the names of known patients with epilepsy. Using this, patient notes were identified and reviewed. Whilst the notes were out, the oppor- tunity was also taken to review the diagnosis and appropriateness of treatment.

Who carried out the audit?

The records review was carried out by one of the partners who had a particular interest in epilepsy.

Results

Of the 54 patients entered as suffering from epilepsy on the manual diagnostic index, the diagnosis was thought to be correct in 51.

Table CS4.1   Reason for patient contact in the last five years

Reason for contact	No. of contacts
A fit	13
Drug review	29
New patient contact	2
Initial diagnosis	4
No clear contact	3
Number seen in *last year*	25

Further results are given in Table CS4.1.

There had been no improvement in the contact rate with patients, and the practice criteria and standards were not being met. Further, the results raised more general questions about the functioning of the repeat prescription system.

Changes resulting from audit

The embarrassing findings of this audit stimulated a series of meetings within the practice. These resulted in:

- a new and more competent protocol for the management of epilepsy care;
- an overhaul of the repeat prescribing system, including a transfer of the system to the new practice computer;
- a decision that partners should update their knowledge of epilepsy management.

Was the audit repeated?

The audit has not been repeated as yet. However, this is clearly an area where continuous audits will be required until the practice can be sure that the new standards are reached and maintained. Future audits of the modified repeat prescription system are planned, to see if it works as intended.

Benefits to practice

- A better standard of care for patients with epilepsy.
- The prospect of improvement in the request for repeat prescriptions.

- The need for new clnical knowledge and skills was identified.
- Improved professional satisfaction for the doctors.

Comment

This audit demonstrates the value of clinical criteria and standards against which subsequent care can be assessed (*see* Chapter 6). It shows also that these criteria and standards are not always implemented by clinicians, a fact which may only be revealed by audit.

As in Case Studies 2 and 3, the practice had management arrangements which enabled the changes identified as necessary actually to be implemented.

Case Study 5

Subject of audit

AN audit of process and intermediate outcome to improve the effectiveness of rubella immunization among adolescent girls within the practice population using practice activity analysis.

Background

For many years, the routine immunization of young females against rubella had been carried out by the medical and nursing staff of the local health authority. The practice had identified several problems arising from this.

1 Information about children immunized was often slow in arriving from the health authority, which meant that the practice records of those patients were incomplete.
2 Some girls were unsure whether they had been immunized.

It became clear that staffing problems at the clinic were causing delays in immunizing; immunization had become a crisis response by the authority to a request from the practice for information about the rubella status of individual patients. The practice team decided to take over the provision of this service, and the recently employed practice nurse was given responsibility for it.

Reason for audit

To ensure that the new practice service was at least as effective as the local authority system.

Aims of audit

The aims were:

- to measure the immunization status of eligible females at 8 months, and 2 years after the installation of the new programme;
- to provide feedback on effectiveness to the practice nurse and partners.

Method

Girls eligible for immunization were identified and sent for using the age–sex register. If a girl failed to respond to two requests, her mother was contacted by telephone and, if possible, the girl was offered another appointment or the reason for non-attendance was discovered and listed.

The practice nurse assessed the results, although it could have been done by any member of the administrative staff.

Results

The results are shown in Table CS5.1.

This audit showed a higher level of uptake in Year 1 than in Year 2, but for both years the uptake was much higher than that achieved by the local health authority. Fear of needles was given as the main reason for refusal.

Table CS5.1

Action	Year 1 (at 8 months)	Year 2
Girls called	51	41
Immunized at surgery	45	36
Immunized at school	2	1
Refused	2	4
Agreed to have immunization later	2	0

Changes resulting from audit

The practice nurse had clear evidence of her effectiveness and the partners were satisfied that the new arrangements were better than immunization through the health authority clinic. No major changes were considered necessary. Nevertheless, the practice formulated a new target: to achieve a 100% immunization rate. The partners chose an ideal standard (*see* Chapter 6) because they recognized that effective protection is person-specific. The practice nurse also sought new strategies to persuade defaulters to be immunized.

Was the audit repeated?

With the advent of computerization in the practice, continuous performance monitoring has been established. The immunization status of girls in the practice list is recorded in the practice nurse's annual report to the partnership. 100% rates have been achieved in two consecutive years.

Comment

This audit shows the relationship between the process of care and its outcome in terms of protection against rubella conferred on patients at risk. It is one of the few situations where an 'ideal standard' is both clinically desirable and achievable *provided that* the practice operates continuous performance monitoring as part of its management function.

Case Study 6

Subject of audit

A process audit attempting to reduce clinical error in the use of H_2-antagonists by case review.

Background

This partnership uses a practice formulary. It was agreed that the H_2-antagonist to be prescribed routinely should be cimetidine.

Reason for audit

PACT data had revealed more prescribing of ranitidine than was agreed by policy. The question was whether there was a noteworthy departure from the practice standard for the prescription of H_2-antagonists, and if so why.

Aim of audit

To review the prescribing patterns of cimetidine and ranitidine and to establish current practice.

Method

Patients on repeat prescriptions for either cimetidine or ranitidine were identified from the data held on the practice computer. In addition, any patient given a prescription for an H_2-antagonist during a consultation was noted.

The manual records of all patients were reviewed and the reasons for prescribing identified.

The objectives of the records review were to:

- determine the pattern of H_2-antagonist use;
- find out whether partners were complying with practice standards which required that:

(a) the preferred practice H_2-antagonist should be cimetidine;
(b) a clear diagnosis of peptic ulcer or hiatus hernia should be achieved before prescribing;
(c) all patients taking H_2-antagonists should be encouraged to take them episodically rather than permanently.

Who carried out the audit?

As clinical data were involved, the records review was carried out by the partners; one partner had responsibility for ensuring the task was completed, and for collating and analysing the data.

Results

In general, the partners felt that there was reasonable compliance with the practice standards.

As an illustration, one partner had 25 patients taking cimetidine, 400 mg; of these, 25 had a proven diagnosis, 7 took episodic treatment, 4 had never been tried off-treatment, 13 had been off-treatment but without long-term success, and 1 had just started treatment.

Another partner had 19 patients taking ranitidine, 150 mg; of these, 16 had a clear diagnosis, 6 took episodic treatment, 8 had never been tried off long-term treatment, 4 had been tried off long-term but without long-term effect, and 1 had died of unrelated illness.

Personal analyses were available for all partners, which could be compared with aggregated results.

Changes resulting from audit

At a clinical meeting to discuss the results, it was decided that:

- it was not necessary to change the formulary;

- the notes of patients who had not been tried off-treatment should be tagged, so that there would be an opportunity to consider episodic treatment in future with their doctor;
- the objective of removing some patients from the hospital follow-up clinics should be pursued.

Was the audit repeated?

Future audits will be performed to check that the standard is still being followed, as part of a regular review of PACT data. Patients attending hospitals for dyspeptic symptoms, and the reasons for them, have been the subject of consequential audit.

Comment

This audit highlighted the amount of work involved in the manual analysis of notes (Chapter 7). If this type of audit is to become routine, partners must train non-medical staff to undertake it.

The audit demonstrated that the discussion and analysis by the partners was inadequate. Although confronted with personal and aggregate data showing apparently significant divergences from their own explicit criteria and standards, they chose to pass over these. This pattern of behaviour can easily go unquestioned unless the practice has an effective system for handling the results of audit and bringing about change (*see* Chapter 10).

Case Study 7

Subject of audit

A process audit demonstrating the standard of care in the practice through the use of a tracer condition, namely hypertension.

Background

A practice team decided to audit its care of patients with hypertension about 10 years ago after which it introduced some criteria for care. The questions considered by the partners were as follows.

- We believe we provide good care for our patients with hypertension. Is that true?
- What standards can be measured?
- Do these provide evidence of good care?
- How does our care compare with defined standards?
- How does my care compare with that of my partners/my peers?
- Can I improve?
- Should I improve?

The original criteria and standards for the care of hypertensives as agreed by the practice are listed below.

- The initial diagnosis should be based on three (minimum) recordings of a diastolic pressure > 100 mmHg.
- There should be a record of:
  urine analysis;
  smoking history;
  family history;
  height and weight.
- The medication should be recorded.
- The current (controlled) diastolic pressure should be < 90 mmHg and should be recorded within the preceding year.

Reason for the audit

A new trainee commented to the partners that she could not reconcile the practice's stated belief that it provided good care for its hypertensive patients with her difficulty in finding information in the notes. The second reason for audit was the death of a 62-year-old man from a cerebrovascular accident who had had, when the notes were perused, a diagnosis of hypertension some 15 years previously. His hypertension had been treated for about 5 years and then lost to follow-up, although there were several entries in the notes about other consultations. These incidents led the practice team to question its perception of hypertensive care and to audit its compliance with the protocols.

Methods

The practice team decided to use hypertension as a tracer condition (*see* Chapter 8) to examine aspects of chronic care. The audit was carried out when the practice had no age–sex register, disease index or computer. Patients with hypertension were identified in three ways:

- when summarizing the clinical records in the practice;
- from repeat prescriptions for anti-hypertensive drugs;
- opportunistically in surgery and by the practice nurse.

This led to the first hypertensive index and a simple disease index.

With the cases identified the practice team drew up a simple data collection form which identified the year of diagnosis, smoking record, urine analysis and other characteristics in which the practice was interested. It was then just a relatively simple clerical task to go through the records and extract the information.

Results of the audit

The results of this audit were disturbing. Although the prevalence rate and the age–sex distribution of hypertension in the practice matched the figures expected, only 32% of patients had three pre-diagnostic diastolic blood pressure measurements taken. On average smoking was recorded in 60% of patients, but there were wide variations among partners in recording; urine analysis was recorded in < 50% of cases, family history in < 15%, height in < 10% and weight in < 15%. Current medication was recorded in 98% of cases; and 80% had a recent diastolic pressure of < 90 mmHg.

The partners felt that if their diagnosis had been correct originally the treatment they were prescribing was reasonably successful. However, this audit did not demonstrate good care as they had previously defined it. It was also obvious that the clinical record keeping was incomplete.

Changes resulting from audit

Discussion of the results led to the following changes.

- Revision of the protocol to include, for example, the measurement of fasting lipids, and an agreement about the drugs to prescribe in hypertension.

- An acceptance of a protocol for the diagnosis and management of patients with hypertension.
- An agreement about what to record.
- The development of a vascular clinic where the practice nurse works to a protocol generated by the doctors.
- Definition of the role of the team in measuring, recording and advising on hypertension.

Was the audit repeated?

A repeat audit has demonstrated that 100% of the hypertensive patients have their smoking and urine analysis recorded, 90% have family history recorded, and 100% have their weight and height recorded. Since the generation of the protocol, all new diagnoses have been based on three diastolic pressure measurements of > 100 mmHg.

Comment

All those involved in health care may have a different perception of good care. For different people, audit can be used to demonstrate different things; to a politician it will have to measure cost effectiveness; to a manager it will have to measure efficiency; to a receptionist possibly punctuality; to a doctor job satisfaction; to a patient, concern, interest, and relief from the illness.

For most audit processes, demonstrating good care often starts with simple questions. In this case, did all patients with the diagnosis of hypertension have a blood pressure recording in the notes in the last year? The pattern of recording data was not originally compatible with good care; there were demonstrable gaps in performance when compared against agreed standards. An improvement in record-keeping was necessary and, as a result, good care and control can now be demonstrated to patients by using computer graphics, computer protocols, and checklists. These also remind partners of the standards previously agreed. Improvement in morbidity or mortality has yet to be demonstrated.

Post script

This audit stimulated the practice team to examine their clinical care in two other areas — asthma and gout. The audit of the treatment of patients with gout showed reasonable doctor compliance with the practice's predetermined standard for the frequency of checking and the target serum level of uric acid to be achieved. However, there were major inter-partner differences in the treatment of asthmatic patients, for example, in the use of peak flow recordings, and the number of different drugs prescribed (42). These variations reflected the fact that the practice had no agreed protocols or standards for the treatment of asthma, and consequently the quality of the medical record-keeping was also variable.

Revised protocols for asthma and gout are now in use, and patients with these conditions are subject to further regular monitoring to ensure partner compliance with agreed protocols and standards.

Case Study 8

Subject of audit

A review of organizational error to establish why supposed improvements in the quality of management within a practice through the appointment of a deputy practice manager, had not achieved the desired results (*see* Chapter 10).

Background

The experience, education and reading of the partners had convinced them that good management at the doctor/patient level normally led to an improvement in clinical care and an increase in the job satisfaction (RCGP, 1985[1]; Fraser, 1987[2]). They believed that improved management in the wider context should result in improvements to the functioning of the partnership and ultimately to better services for patients (Drury, 1990)[3].

A practice manager was appointed in 1983 in response to an increasingly complex administrative burden. The person appointed was computer-literate, the ex-personnel manager of a large hotel, who also ran the financial side of a small business. The new practice manager was left to develop the practice and her own role within it.

Five years later, the size and complexity of the practice had increased. Consequently, the practice manager had become increasingly busy. She had attended several courses on practice management and was anxious to extend her role in the development of the practice and its quality of care. To achieve these objectives, she proposed to the partners that a deputy practice manager be appointed to take over the routine administration of the practice, so that she could be released to obtain further training through an Open University course, and participate more in the strategic management of the practice, including the preparation for fund-holding.

A deputy practice manager was appointed, who had experience of managing people and finance.

Reason for the audit

Initially, the new appointment seemed to work well. However, the practice manager became busier. She was still administering the practice, trying to teach the deputy and the course work was beginning to arrive in quantity. Unfortunately, three months after the appointment of the deputy practice manager, the practice manager went on sick leave with a disabling physical condition.

The partnership turned to the deputy practice manager to take over. However, it became apparent that the practice manager was the only person who knew how to run the practice. The partners realized that having a deputy practice manager did not ensure continuity of quality of management, nor did it provide the enhanced management input that they had expected. They decided to identify the main organizational areas of the practice and delegate them to specific partners who had the power to make an executive decision in each area.

The partners met regularly to make management decisions on behalf of the absent practice manager, and it was decided that this approach would be more efficient than unstructured management meetings. It mirrored the way the partners had dealt with clinical policy decisions for years: one partner delegated to research a particular clinical area brought his/her ideas for discussion with the other partners to agree a clinical protocol had been devised after appropriate partnership discussion.

The deputy practice manager returned to her previous job. The partners took the opportunity to investigate whether the post of deputy practice manager is able to provide an improvement in the quality of practice management.

Aim of the audit

To review the existing management structure and to assess it against the management needs of the practice.

Method

The original aims of the appointment of a deputy practice manager were re-examined and a chart showing the current organization was drawn. The roles played by the partners, the practice manager and the other staff in the decision to appoint a deputy practice manager were also examined.

Who carried out the audit?

Owing to the fundamental nature of the audit, it was undertaken by all partners with the support of the existing practice manager.

Results

The basic finding was that the responsibilities of the deputy practice manager post had not been thought about by anyone other than the practice manager. Each of the partners and members of staff had different perceptions of the role of deputy practice manager and of the practice manager herself.

It was also clear that the partnership decicion-making process was inadequate; a considerable amount of the practice manager's time was spent on trying to obtain appropriate decisions. Either the practice manager made decisions on her own, or was forced to present issues to all of the partners which took time. Initially, the partners had not delegated to each other responsibility for particular parts of practice organization; this would have given the practice manager points of reference for specific areas of practice organization, and helped the decision-making process. It would then have been possible to identify the range of decisions that could be made by the practice manager alone, by the practice manager and the relevant partner, and by the whole partnership.

The problems that led to the failure of achieving the stated objectives in appointing a deputy practice manager were as follows.

- Poor communication and decision-making mechanisms at partnership level.
- Inexperience and poor training of the deputy practice manager in the practical aspects of the functioning of the practice.
- The demography of the practice — two large health centres led to duplication of effort in the implementation of policies.
- Unrealistic expectations of the deputy practice manager post among staff and partners.

Changes resulting from audit

Areas of activity

Key areas of practice managerial activity were identified as follows.

- Access and communication.
- Buildings.
- Education.
- Emergencies and out of hours.
- Equipment and computers.
- Finance and fund-holding.
- Prescribing.
- Preventive care.
- Referral patterns.
- Staff recruitment and training.
- Teamwork and extracurricular activities.
- The Contract.

These areas were assigned to each of the partners who had the executive power to make a decision in that area on behalf of the partnership whilst regularly reporting to the partnership on progress.

Two of the existing practice secretaries had applied for the post of deputy practice manager, having been on a local AMSPAR course. It was proposed to appoint them as office managers, one at each health centre. By splitting their existing jobs and appointing part-time secretaries to fill the secretarial gaps left by their redeployment, the practice was able to present the changes to the FHSA as a no-cost option, whilst staffing levels remained unchanged. This strategy ensured that both office managers had experience and knowledge of the functioning of the practice. The agreed list of management areas within the practice was divided between the office managers, and it was clear which partner to consult in case of problems and which office manager. All were encouraged to share so that absence did not mean the practice would be without effective management.

Figure CS8.1

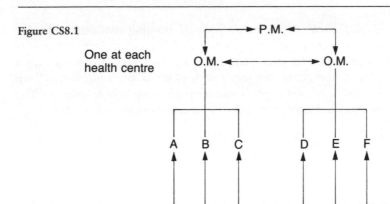

One at each
health centre

Key
A   Teamwork/Communication
B   Finance, Fund-holding/Referrals
C   Equipment, Computers/Out of Hours
D   The Contract/Preventive care
E   Education (the trainee)/Prescribing
F   Staff/Buildings
P.M. Practice manager
O.M. Office manager
The partners are represented by the numbers 1–6.

The new management structure is shown in Fig. CS8.1.

Development plan

When the practice manager returned to work her first task was to produce a practice development plan in preparation for fund-holding status. This she was able to do because the responsibility for daily operational management had been delegated to the office managers and the relevant partners. She discussed her plans at length with the relevant partners, particularly those responsible for fund-holding and staff, and the two office managers. They quickly identified all potential problems with regard to space, staff rotas and the long-term relationship between the fund-holding staff and permanent staff. Appropriate appointments were made in record time.

Practice management

The benefits of the practice manager's Open University course also became apparent. The practice manager and office managers began to meet weekly to plan and implement office policies. Staff training assumed a higher priority, and staff were enrolled in local training courses. Delegation was encouraged, and staff were involved in solving their own problems rather than presenting the practice manager with a series of complaints. Each member of staff was offered a new contract with better job definitions. The use of information technology within the practice began to improve.

Was the audit repeated?

The audit was not repeated. However, regular performance monitoring has now been built in as part of the management cycle (*see* Chapter 10).

Comment

By tracing the contributing factors to a management action by the partners, this audit revealed not only whether the desired end had been achieved (which it had not), but also whether the management processes were effective. Audit allowed the identification of an organizational error, i.e. the provision of a deputy practice manager, and alternative solutions could be introduced once the problem had been evaluated. This Case Study demonstrates how effective an audit of process can be in changing organizations.

Case Study 9

Subject of audit

A process audit to identify whether opportunistic screening is the most effective method of ensuring that patients between the ages of 20 and 80 years have their blood pressure recorded in every 5-year period.

Background

In 1981, this practice of 5 partners and 10 500 patients appointed a specially trained practice nurse to screen for raised blood pressure. Of those aged between 40 and 65 years, 84% responded to a direct invitation for a blood-pressure check. In 1986, it was found that most patients had not had their blood pressure taken since the initial recording. The practice policy on hypertension was changed in that year following a literature review. A new practice criterion stated that all patients between the ages of 20 and 80 years should have their blood pressure measured every five years (Petrie et al., 1986[1]; Swales et al., 1989).[2]

As the practice was unable to devote sufficient nurse time to a systematic re-screening, it was decided to screen the relevant practice population opportunistically during routine surgery consultations (Hart, 1970, 1987[3,4]). All the records were clearly stamped to remind the doctors to record the blood pressure (plus alcohol, smoking habit and weight) during future surgery consultations.

The experience of the systematic screening programme in 1981 had shown that direct invitations needed to take account of work and life-style patterns. Working men responded best to evening appointments, whereas young women responded best to morning appointments.

Reason for the audit

After four years, there were still some patients attending surgery who had not had their blood pressure recorded. Whereas, at the beginning of 1987, virtually every patient needed a blood pressure check, by 1990 a large percentage of patients attending had an appropriately dated blood pressure measurement in the notes. The degree of doctor alertness needed to record blood pressure and to update the records was therefore lower.

Other changes had taken place in the practice: in particular, a computer had been installed and the number of practice nurses had increased. The use of the practice nurses was proving to be popular with patients in line with the experience of others (Jewell and Hope, 1988[5]).

Aims of the audit

1 To assess the efficiency of the opportunistic screening programme by identifying those patients between the ages of 20 and 80 years who had

an appropriately dated blood pressure measurement taken within the previous 4 years.

2 To improve the effectiveness of the opportunistic screening programme by examining the ages and sex of those who had not had a blood pressure measurement taken in the last 4 years, with a view to inviting them to a nurse-run clinic for a blood pressure reading, and giving appointments tailored to their assumed work pattern.

Methods

The audit was carried out in only one of the two health centres which served a population of 4100 people.

Two computer programmes were devised: the first counted those patients between 20 and 80 years who had had their blood pressure measured in the last 5 years; the second programme made an age–sex histogram over the same time-scale of those patients in the same age-group who had not had their blood pressure measured.

Who carried out the audit?

The computer programme was devised by one of the partners. Data entry was carried out by the reception staff. As there had been no computer in the practice at the beginning of the data collection, there was a backlog of many hundreds of blood pressure readings to be entered before the audit could take place.

Once the backlog of data had been cleared, the doctors were responsible for inputting measurements at surgery contact, and nurses and reception staff for contact elsewhere in the health centre. Enthusiasm was maintained by giving progress reports to those who measured blood pressure opportunistically; the production of these reports exerted peer pressure, especially when it was clear that a certain partner was not conforming to the agreed data-entry protocol.

Results

The distribution by age and sex of patients who had their blood pressure recorded in the past 5 years is shown in Table CS9.1.

Table CS9.1 To show numbers of patients between the ages of 20 and 80 years who have had BP recorded in the last 5 years

Opportunistic screening
(of 4100 patients)

Sex	Number	With/without (BP record)	With/without (per cent)
Male	1334	989/345	74/26
Female	1288	1100/188	85/15
Both	2622	2089/533	80/20

Analysis showed that more than 20% of the target population had not had blood pressure recorded in the last 5 years. The age–sex histogram (Table CS9.2) of those without a blood pressure reading showed a preponderance of men, possibly because women not only attend more frequently as a group, but also have their blood pressure recorded during attendance for oral contraception and/or antenatal care.

Changes resulting from audit

Towards the end of the first 5-year period, so few patients were attending surgery who had not had their blood pressure recorded it suggested that

Table CS9.2 Age–sex histogram of patients between the ages of 20 and 80 years who have not had BP recorded in the last 5 years

Opportunistic screening
(of 4100 patients)

All	Male	Female	Male	Age bands (years)	Female
5	0	5	* *	80–84	*
19	9	10	*	75–79	* *
17	4	13	* * *	70–74	* * *
22	13	9	* * *	65–69	* *
20	12	8	* * * *	60–64	* *
25	14	11	* * * * * * *	55–59	* * *
40	27	13	* * * * *	50–54	* * *
40	21	19	* * * * * * * *	45–49	* * * * *
47	33	14	* * * * * * * *	40–44	* * *
45	29	16	* * * * * * * *	35–39	* * * *
57	34	23	* * * * * * * * * * * * * *	30–34	* * * * *
89	68	21	* * * * * * * * * * * * * * * * * * * *	25–29	* * * * *
107	81	26		20–24	* * * * * *
533	345	188			

little impact could be made on the 20% who still had to have blood pressure measured if opportunistic recording continued alone. It was decided to continue opportunistic screening, but direct invitations to attend a practice nurse-run clinic would also be sent to patients who had not had their blood pressure recorded. Men aged between 20 and 60 years and women aged between 40 and 75 years were sent an evening appointment; men aged between 60 and 75 years and women aged between 20 and 40 years were sent a morning appointment.

The letters were sent using a modification of the computer programme used to generate the age–sex histogram combined with the facility of the computer to generate pre-defined letters.

In addition, all patients over the age of 75 years were to have their blood pressure measured by the district nurses as part of the New Contract arrangements.

Was the audit repeated?

Although this new strategy is an ongoing process, an audit of uptake to date suggests that at the end of the current 5-year period, 88% of the target population will have had their blood pressure recorded. Different strategies will have to be devised at the end of the 5-year period to improve on the overall uptake during the next 5-year cycle.

Thoughts on data handling

Entering a mass of data can be harmful to staff harmony; the practice team listed some 'dos and don'ts' and these are shown in Fig. CS9.1.

Data entry presents two main problem areas. One is standardization and the other is volume (*see* Chapter 5). Data must be entered into the computer in the same form by everyone. Standardization involved a meeting of those who were to enter the data with someone who demonstrated to the staff that confusion and time wasting would arise if standardization was not agreed.

Comment

Raised blood pressure is a symptomless condition worth detecting as its treatment is of proven value in reducing mortality from strokes by 45%,

Figure CS9.1

WHAT TO DO

DO   Involve the staff in understanding the reasons for the data entry.
DO   Create realistic targets with the help of the staff.
DO   Be flexible about finishing dates (but keep them firmly in sight).
DO   Listen to staff difficulties about time and space and facilitate solutions.
DO   Meet to assess progress, listen to problems and motivate.
DO   Ensure the staff can enter data correctly.

WHAT NOT TO DO

DON'T   Issue orders to complete the task within a specific time-scale.
DON'T   Assume the staff can tackle a mountain of work without the creation of a lot of tension and resentment.
DON'T   Become dependent upon one member of staff (data entry can be tedious, and sickness and retirement will lead to confusion and delay).
DON'T   Dictate the mechanics of data entry (the staff can do this).

and mildly raised blood pressure is a risk factor for the development of ischaemic heart disease (MRC, 1985).[6]

Before treatment can be initiated, hypertension has to be detected. As most people are registered with a general practitioner, and 90% of patients consult their general practitioner within a 5-year period, general practice is the best place to detect and monitor patients with raised blood pressure.

The detection of raised blood pressure in general practice patients has been attempted by systemic screening of a total practice population (De Souza et al., 1976[7]) and by opportunistic case finding (Hart, 1970[3]). A combination of the two methods is probably ideal, by sending an invitation to those who have not had their blood pressure recorded opportunistically in a 5-year period.

This audit encompassed three necessary components: an objective whose value was based on published evidence, a method of comparing actual and stated performance and strategies to improve actual performance.

The final audit of blood pressure screening will have to review the effects on morbidity and mortality from stroke and ischaemic heart disease of identifying and trying to reduce a common risk factor — increased blood pressure. It will be many years before the practice team can measure such trends. It is likely, however, that the routine use of medical audit will be one of the most powerful tools at the disposal of general practice in improving the quality of care necessary to achieve this outcome.

Much was learned in the process about data entry. There are two main problem areas: standardization and volume. Data has to be entered into the computer in a standard form. To ensure standardization a meeting was held of those who were to enter the data, and one person was responsible for demonstrating that confusion, time wastage and inadequate results would arise if standardization was not achieved.

This audit demonstrates the contribution a computer can make to patient care. There are few manual search systems that will rapidly identify patients who have not attended for a particular service or measurement, especially when the number of patients is large, whereas computers can perform this task easily (these particular programmes take about 45 minutes to run).

Case Study 10

Subject of audit

To identify the reasons for frustration and irritation within a practice, and enhance professional satisfaction.

Background

This practice comprised four partners (three male and one female); there were about 8500 patients registered, and the practice operated from a health authority clinic. The partners employed a senior receptionist/practice manager, a secretary, a part-time nurse and six part-time receptionists. A community nurse, a health visitor and a midwife were attached to the practice, but accountable to their own nursing hierarchies. The senior receptionist/practice manager had recently retired, and there was a new practice manager who had a commercial background, which was deemed important as the partners wanted to re-appraise their management systems to ensure they met targets, maximized income, and improved patient care.

Reason for the audit

The practice manager felt it was not possible for him to make any changes within the organization without a clear understanding of the reasons for the feelings of frustration, irritation and low morale exhibited by the practice team.

Aims of audit

To identify the reasons for the malaise within the practice, and to offer a range of solutions.

Methods

1 Practice activity analysis. The practice manager set up systems for collected data on attendances at surgeries and clinics, recording home visits and carrying out random checks comparing times of appointment against times patients were actually seen, by partner or by nurse.

   The partners looked at FHSA returns on cervical cytology and pre-school immunizations, and the practice manager assessed the availability of information on the rubella status of females in the practice, the monitoring of hypertension, and the over-75s screening programme.
2 Patient satisfaction survey. A survey of patient satisfaction was carried out after each consultation and consisted of a simple questionnaire (see Fig. CS10.1).

Figure CS10.1 Patient survey

1. These questions relate specifically to the consultation that you have just had.
   (i)   Did you see the doctor of your preferred choice?
         Yes/No
   (ii) Were you able to make this appointment for a time that suited you?
         Yes/No
   (iii) The length of time the consultation lasted was:
         (a) Too short to allow me to explain my problem.
   or   (b) Reasonable but I would have preferred longer.
   or   (c) About right.
   (iv) Were you seen promptly on your appointment time?
         Yes/No
   If your answer is No, then please answer the next questions:
   (v)   Did you have to wait up to 10 minutes?
         Did you have to wait more than 15 minutes?
         Did you have to wait more than 30 minutes?

The last question relates to the service the practice provides:
2. Overall, are you satisfied with the care and attention you get from the doctors and staff in the practice?
Yes/No/Don't know

Table CS10.1 Consultation and referral rate

Doctor	Total surgery consultations	Doctor initiated consultations (%)	Extras (unlisted) (%)	Total home visits	Repeat visits (%)	'Clinic' consultations	Total patients seen	No. hospital referrals
Dr A	1241	36	10	256	27	349	1846	30
Dr B	1302	33	9	378	32	–	1680	36
Dr C	1291	25	12	357	19	323	1651	58
Dr D	1309	36	12	257	25	–	1566	34
Total	5143			1248		672	7063	158

Quarter 1 July–30 September
Consultation rate = 3.2
Referral rate = 75 per 1000 patients/year

3 A confidential enquiry was made to each member of staff. They had to write a brief description of their job as they understood it to be, including all the tasks they were expected to do, describe (in absolute confidence) things that made the job more difficult than it need be, and identify any further training needs, and what training they would like the practice to provide.

Who carried out the audit?

The audit was largely carried out under the direction of the practice manager who was released from other duties for three months. Reception staff collected most of the data, and the partners encouraged patients to fill in the patient satisfaction survey.

Results

1 Practice activity analysis. An extract from data on consultation and hospital referral patterns, as part of the practice activity analysis, is shown in Table CS10.1. An extract from the immunization data collected is shown in Table CS10.2.

Table CS10.2 Immunization rates

Children aged 2 years or under on the 1st of the (relevant) quarter.
Group I: Diphtheria, Tetanus and Polio (3 doses)
    78% of target population

Group II: Pertussis (3 doses)
    45% of target population

Group III: Measles (1 dose)
         or MMR
    69% of target population
NB: The local authority clinic had carried out 70% of these completed courses.

Children aged 5 years on 1st of the (relevant) quarter.
Pre-school booster targets.
    76% of target population.
NB: The local authority clinic had carried out 95% of these.

Hypertension/smoking recording. Despite a declared policy of measuring blood pressure in all patients in the age-group 40–65 years at least every 5 years, a random survey of 1 in 10 records from the survey population showed < 50% had had their blood pressure recorded.

The results were similar when the recording of smoking habit was examined; < 50% of the records surveyed did not indicate whether the patient smoked.

2 Patient satisfaction survey. The results confirmed the suspicions of the practice that their poor timekeeping and inadequate appointment system were having an adverse effect on their relationships with their patients. However, the results from the general satisfaction question were encouraging and showed that the practice still had a positive image.

3 Staff enquiry. Information from the enquiry and interviews with the staff showed that the practice was not employing its full quota of reimbursable staff. The practice nurse felt she had neither the time nor the skills to make an appropriate contribution to the work of the practice. The employed staff had not been informed or consulted about any changes that were taking place; in particular, they felt threatened by the appointment of the practice manager.

In more general terms, the following deficiencies were identified in the practice.

- There was no common goal or purpose.
- There were no clinical protocols.
- The organization of the practice was inappropriate.
- There were no appraisals of performance.
- There was no recognition of training needs, nor any provision for meeting them.
- There was a dearth of good basic data regularly available.

Changes resulting from audit

The changes can be summarized as follows.

1 The practice started to have regular practice meetings with an agenda and minutes.
2 The partners began to develop an agreed and written common purpose or goal.
3 The organizational structure of the practice was reviewed.
4 A clear definition of the relationships and responsibilities within the practice, particularly those between the practice manager and the doctors, was agreed.

5 Staff appraisals were introduced, based on new and agreed job descriptions.
6 A training programme for doctors and staff was set up: priority and resources were set aside for skills training for the practice nurse, and management training for one of the partners.
7 A series of practice meetings was instituted to discuss the production of clinical protocols.
8 The staff complement was increased.
9 More time was allocated for surgeries and individual consultations.

Was the audit repeated?

This overall audit was not repeated, but a series of more specific audits were instituted to ensure the practice team achieves its objectives in the key areas identified.

Comment

This case study demonstrated how an audit can be used to discover what is creating the frustration, irritation and inefficiency in a practice. Such an audit can be achieved only by the injection of a new resource; in this case, the new practice manager was given 3 months to investigate the problem, without which an external consultant would probably have had to have been employed to identify the solutions.

Case Study 11

Subject of audit

A process audit to reduce clinical and organizational error, using the confidential case enquiry method of audit.

Background

Mr and Mrs Black, their son Kevin (aged 5 years) and daughter Tracey (aged 1 year), had originally registered with the practice two years ago. Mr Black had been a labourer until recently, but was now out of work. Mrs Black was a state enrolled nurse.

All the Blacks had active medical problems. Mr Black had chronic asthma, a condition for which he consulted Dr Adam regularly. Mrs Black had a longstanding history of undiagnosed, episodic abdominal pain, complicated by bouts of vomiting, especially in the evenings. She had seen Dr Baker regularly but, despite extensive investigation, no firm diagnosis had been established. When bouts of vomiting occurred, the only intervention that gave reasonably prompt and symptomatic relief was intramuscular metaclopropamide. Kevin was subject to recurrent earache and had recently had grommets inserted. Tracey had recently been diagnosed as suffering from an allergy to cow's milk. When the children became ill, Mrs Black tended to take them to see the doctor most readily available.

One evening, Kevin had a further attack of earache and Dr Edwards visited him at home. Dr Edwards found no serious abnormality and advised no medication. Kevin appeared comfortable.

The following day, Mr and Mrs Black took Kevin to hospital for a checkup on the grommets. They were told that one eardrum was inflamed, and that an antibiotic was indicated. Later that day, Mrs Black attended surgery with Tracey, when she saw Dr Collins. She asked Dr Collins how she could make a complaint about Dr Edwards who, she said, had failed to prescribe an antibiotic when the hospital doctor had said it was necessary. Dr Collins told Dr Edwards of the problem.

Reason for the audit

Dr Edwards was somewhat surprised by the complaint, because he had judged the child to be only slightly unwell and, as far as he could learn from Dr Baker, that was still the case. He decided to follow up the complaint with the parents, to see if he could find out what the problem really was, what seemed to have gone wrong, and to try and restore relationships.

He visited the parents, and during the course of the discussion (see below) it became clear that a more detailed enquiry, involving the management of all the members of the family, would be appropriate, i.e. a confidential case audit was indicated.

Aims of audit

The purpose of the case audit was to define the family's concerns with particular regard to alleged clinical mismanagement. It would also try and establish what the family expected of the practice.

Method

In this confidential case enquiry, the following steps were taken.

1 An interview with the complainants.
2 A review of the case notes.
3 Recording the findings.
4 Discussion of the findings, leading to conclusions, with partners and patients (separately).

Who carried out the audit?

The audit was carried out by Dr Edwards as a continuation of his initial visit.

Results

The interview with the patients took just over 1 hour. The principal findings of fact were as follows.

1 The family had moved to this practice because of dissatisfaction with their previous practice. They were dismayed to find that in some respects the care they had received in this practice had not been of the standard they had expected.
2 Mr and Mrs Black thought that Dr Edwards, who had attended Kevin promptly, had been cursory in his examination and brief in his discussion of the problem.
3 Mrs Black was unhappy about the treatment she received for her sickness and abdominal pain when symptoms presented out of hours, and when a partner other than Dr Baker came.
    "I'm never right until I get some Maxalon, and I shouldn't have to say that every time."

Nevertheless, she liked Dr Baker, had confidence in her, and wished only that there could be better communication between Dr Baker and the other partners about the management of Mrs Black in an emergency.

4 Both parents thought that Dr Collins should have diagnosed Tracey's milk allergy sooner.

5 Mr Black said that he was very satisfied with Dr Adam's treatment of his asthma.

6 There seemed to be no good reason, other than parental convenience, why the children tended to be taken to any partner, rather than the partner with whom the child was registered.

Mr Black, commenting on the practice, said that in the main he and his wife were satisfied with their care but they were surprised that the care could easily become less satisfactory in patches.

"Surely you must have some systems for dealing with families like us who have more than one problem on the go at once."

The essential findings from this interview were passed to the other partners. The second stage of the audit began with a review of the case notes of all the family members. The case notes describing the management of both Mr and Mrs Black were considered to be full and appropriate, each giving a coherent account of their problems, the working diagnoses, and the management plans, including up-to-date drug treatment. The case notes for the children were more brief, revealed multiple partner entries, and underlined the parent's impression of discontinuity leading, in Tracey's case, to delay in diagnosis, and, in Kevin's case, to conflicting advice on the management of the ear condition.

In the opinion of the partners, the interview and case notes review had shown that the parents' initial complaint about Dr Edwards was a token presentation of an underlying problem, rather than a reflection of a serious single error. Seen in that way, the complaint was basically justified. Problems of continuity and communication were revealed that reflected deficiencies in the practice's systems, and therefore such problems could recur.

Changes resulting from audit

Changes were grouped under three main headings.

1 For the Black family. To improve continuity of care for the children, Mr and Mrs Black agreed with the partners on the following.

- Both children would be re-registered with Dr Baker. When Dr Baker was unavailable, the first alternative would be Dr Adams.

- All partners were fully briefed by Dr Baker on Mrs Black's problem with abdominal pain, and how best to manage it.
- The focus on two doctors for the family (rather than one which might have been considered ideal) reflected the desire of both Mr Black and Mrs Black to keep their 'own doctor', that is Dr Adams and Dr Baker.

2 Impact on practice systems. The case raised several questions about practice systems, especially those bearing on continuity. These are now being considered further by the practice manager, and supplementary audits may be performed.

3 For the audit procedure. The case prompted further discussion amongst the partners about the value of auditing critical incidents. Two points were made. The question of who should be responsible for such audits was raised. In this instance, the benefits of the person about whom the complaint had been made were traded against the potential lack of objectivity which could result through personal involvement. There seemed to be no easy answer. In principle, it was felt that an uninvolved partner would be best placed to conduct such enquiries whenever possible.

Second, the method should have included formal interviews with the partners concerned about their particular contributions to the family's care; ideally, this should have involved the relevant hospital doctors.

Comment

It is often said that an effective audit cannot be carried out on one case. However, this case study illustrates that this is untrue if the yardstick is to be change resulting in an improvement in care both for the individual patient and more generally. This form of audit represents excellent value for money, in that the circumstances that provoke it are likely to result in change. There are no complicated data to collect, no difficult analyses to be made, and no expense to be incurred other than the time and care involved in the examination itself.

Confidential case enquiries are threatening because they involve an exploration of probable error. It is unlikely that the partners in this case would have consented to this kind of audit unless there had been prior agreement that such a method would be used and the results would be kept confidential within the practice. This case study helps to illustrate the general points about the handling of confidential case enquiries described in Chapter 8.

Case Study 12

Subject of audit

AUDIT of process and outcome assessing the effectiveness of a changed approach to the delivery of diabetic care.

Background

In 1985, a practice was concerned about its delivery of diabetic care. It was decided to set up a diabetic clinic, to identify and register all diagnosed diabetic patients, and provide a framework of care for those not attending hospital clinics.

The practice compiled a diabetic register, produced guidelines for care in the form of a protocol, established a team for diabetic care and identified the roles of the members of the team — the practice nurse was given lead responsibility.

Reason for the audit

After four years' experience, the practice recognized that they had never tested whether the setting up of the diabetic clinic had led to improved patient care. Considerably more resources were being put into the management of this particular condition with no evidence to show that patient care had improved.

Aims of audit

To test whether the establishment of the diabetic clinic had led to improved patient care, in terms of improved patient education about the condition, better control of the disease and the effective use of formal nursing input.

Method

As an audit-friendly format for patient records had been used from the outset, a simple, record-based audit could be carried out. The following were regarded as essential for the recorded data.

- Date the patient was last seen.
- Whether the patient received GP or hospital care.
- Whether the patient received insulin.
- The patient's current drug therapy.
- Data and result of patient's last:

> eye test;
> foot examinations/advice/chiropody;
> blood pressure;
> smoking history;
> weight/body mass index;
> urine analysis for proteins;
> glycosylated protein estimation.

Who carried out the audit?

The audit was carried out by the practice nurse responsible for the diabetic clinic, with considerable help from the computer operator who carried out the clinical record search.

Results

A comparison of the results in 1985 with those of 1989 is shown in Table CS12.1.

Table CS12.1 Number of patients with diabetes in the practice

	1985	1989
Total patients[1]	156	179
Recorded prevalence (%)	1.1	1.25
Number on insulin (%)	63 (40)	64 (36)
Practice only patients (%)[2]	92 (59)	110 (61)

Notes: [1] All patients of the practice with diabetes
       [2] Practice patients with diabetes looked after by the practice alone

Table CS12.2   Practice patients with diabetes looked after by the practice team alone

	1985	1989
Practice only patients (%)	92 (59)	110 (61)
Number (%) seen in previous 12 months for diabetes	91 (99)	107 (97)
Number with recorded eye tests in previous 12 months	26 (28)	92 (84)
Number with recorded feet examinations/advice/ chiropody provided	No	88 (80)
Number with recorded BP in previous 12 months (%)	records 22 (23)	99 (90)
Number with smoking history recorded	19 (21)	94 (85)
Number with glycosylated protein in previous 12 months (%)	Rarely done	85 (77)

Of the 110 patients currently cared for by the practice team exclusively, 93 regularly attended the diabetic clinic; for these patients, the recording of data was almost 100% (*see* Table CS12.2). The remaining patients were mainly house-bound or in sheltered housing; for them, the level of recording by the doctors was not as comprehensive as for patients attending the clinic.

The results about control were self-evident; there was more systematic recording of data concerned with control.

In addition, the doctors identified six areas that had been contributed to the success of the diabetic care clinic.

1 Clear objectives had been established: to identify and register all the patients with diabetes and to provide a framework for care for those patients not attending the hospital clinic.
2 In terms of identifying patients, the disease register was essential, especially for planning appointments, special checks and for audit. Initially, the practice had been able to identify 156 patients, a prevalence rate of 1.1%. The patient list was held on computer and the practice nurse was responsible for its maintenance. This had worked well.
3 Seeing and recalling patients. The separate diabetic clinic allowed better liaison with the nurse, and a new protocol was devised together with a new record sheet. All patients were given a personal record booklet which gave useful educational information. The nurse was recognized as the key worker, but patients could see their own doctor when required, and had an appointment at least annually for a medical review including an eye examination. The audit demonstrated that patients prefer to receive their next appointment when attending a clinic; the computer was helpful in identifying the occasional persistent non-attender, and for search and recall for the annual eye test.
4 An audit-friendly records format which generated simple results tables.

5 A functional team. The use of the practice nurse had been demonstrated to be invaluable. She had been able to refer directly to dieticians and chiropodists without consulting the doctors, and a constructive framework for future cooperation had been established.
6 Educating the health professionals. The continued training of the practice nurse had been beneficial. The doctors also attended diabetes symposia and subscribed to a practical journal on diabetes.

Changes resulting from audit

The audit showed that the decision to run a diabetic clinic had been justified. The future requirement for change would be concerned with fine tuning only.

Was the audit repeated?

An annual review of the figures was instituted as part of the normal management process.

Comment

This audit demonstrates the value of using an audit-friendly format for clinical records (*see* Chapter 7), so that data can be abstracted and analysed easily by non-medical practice staff. It also illustrates the value of repeated audit so that change over time can be demonstrated adequately.

Case Study 13

Subject of audit

PROCESS audit assessing patterns of referral practice, through using practice activity analysis (*see* Chapter 7).

Background

This prospective audit was carried out in a practice with 6 partners in an urban area. In the same town, there was a district general hospital with casuality facilities. Moreover, the town was only 14 miles from full regional facilities with a good road link, and from which a number of visiting consultants came for out-patient clinics including paediatrics, dermatology and radiotherapy.

Reason for audit

A new trainee in the practice had a particular interest in referral rates, having just read an article in the *Journal of the Royal College of General Practitioners* (Wilkin and Smith, 1987[1]). The practice was anxious that self-audit/peer view and discussion should help to reveal why referral decisions were made, and establishing an idea of current patterns would be the first step.

Aims of audit

The aim was to document the broad pattern of referrals by specialty and partner.

Method

A simple data collection sheet was devised, to be completed each time a referral letter was signed during November 1989. The limitation of measuring referral rates over a short period of time was recognized, particularly against a background of random fluctuation in patients presenting and requiring referral. The information collected included the sex and age of patient, the hospital, specialty and consultant to whom the patient was referred, an indication of the urgency and the presumptive diagnosis or presenting problem. The reason(s) for referral were indicated with the choice from the following:

- set procedure;
- known diagnosis and/or help with management;
- investigation;

- diagnosis;
- doctor relief.

Who carried out the audit?

The trainee devised and supervised the collection of data and its analysis; individual partners assisted by entering the data for their own referrals on the questionnaire provided. The practice secretaries, who typed the referral letters, reminded doctors if the questionnaire was not completed.

Results

There was a total of 164 referrals over 1 month. The referral rates by doctor and by specialty are shown in Table CS13.1. The numbers of routine and urgent referrals by doctors are shown in Table CS13.2. The numbers of referrals of male and female patients are shown in Table CS13.3. The number of referrals within each referral category are shown in Table CS13.4. Doctors 1–5 were five of the six practice partners, the sixth being

Table CS13.1   Referral rates by doctor and by specialty

Specialty	Doctor							Total
	1	2	3	4	5	6	7	
Obstetrics & Gynaecology	1	2	17	1	1	2	3	27
Surgery	2	3	5	2	5	2	3	21
Orthopaedics	2	0	2	6	2	1	3	16
Physiotherapy	3	0	2	3	4	1	3	16
Ophthalmology	0	3	4	1	2	2	1	13
General medicine	1	2	0	3	2	1	3	12
ENT	2	1	3	2	0	1	1	10
Dermatology	1	1	2	2	2	0	1	9
Paediatrics (inc. surgery)	0	1	2	0	1	1	3	8
Psychiatry (inc. CPNs)	2	1	2	0	2	0	1	8
Other	3	2	8	5	5	1	0	24
Total	17	16	47	25	26	12	21	164
Referral rate/100 consultations	2.5	3.7	7.4	2.9	3.3	1.6	3.6	

Average for practice 3.57

Table CS13.2   Numbers of routine and urgent referrals*

	Doctor							Total
	1	2	3	4	5	6	7	
Urgent	1	1	13	5	1	3	3	27
Routine	16	15	34	18	24	9	18	134
Unspecified	0	0	0	2	1	0	0	3

*Emergency referrals not included as data collected indicated doctor with whom registered rather than referring doctor.

Table CS13.3   Number of referrals of male and female patients

Sex	Doctor							Total
	1	2	3	4	5	6	7	
Male	5	5	5	15	8	10	12	60
Female	5	11	42	10	18	2	9	97
Not specified	7	0	0	0	0	0	0	7

Table CS13.4   Number of referrals within each referral category

Reason for Referral	Doctor							Total
	1	2	3	4	5	6	7	
Set procedure	4	2	11	3	7	2	1	30
Help with management	10	4	21	13	8	7	9	72
Investigation	1	2	5	6	3	0	8	25
Diagnosis	2	9	12	3	8	3	5	42
Doctor relief	1	1	2	0	0	1	0	5

away on a sabbatical; doctor 6 was a locum and doctor 7 was a vocational trainee.

One of the most striking results was the high number of gynaecological referrals, of which 63% had been referred by the one female partner (No. 5); 37.5% of the orthopeadic referrals were made by partner No. 4 who had a particular interest in rheumatology.

Given that the numbers were small, the results tended to suggest that although there was a fairly marked difference in referral rates by individual partners within the practice, putative reasons for the differences, including the types of patients consulting particular doctors with specific problems, could include the sex, age, personality and experience of the doctors concerned. The personality and experience of the doctors may also have a direct influence on referral behaviour.

The high percentage of gynaecological referrals made by the female doctor, and of orthopaedic referrals made by doctor No. 4, reflects the special interests within the practice. Experience in a particular specialty leads to a higher rate of referral to that specialty.

Changes resulting from audit

The audit revealed some patterns and trends in referral patterns that could be pursued. It stimulated discussion on the possibility of reducing unnecessary referrals to hospital clinics by adopting referral between partners.

Was the audit repeated?

The practice is planning further work on referrals.

1 To develop a minimum data set on hospital referrals.
2 The prospective examination of a sample of records, together with doctor interviews, to discover more about the factors that influence a doctors' decision to refer.
3 To try and develop explicit criteria for referral.

Comment

The value of this exploratory audit lies in the further questions it raised amongst the partners about hospital referrals. It demonstrates the value of a short-term, exploratory approach, gathering data sufficient to test the data collection instruments before further use.

Practice activity analysis audits involving short-term data collection and analysis are particularly suitable projects for trainees since they can be completed within their relatively short period of attachment to a practice.

Case Study 14

Subject of audit

IMPROVING the effectiveness and efficiency of rubella immunization using a process audit.

Background

Rubella infection during pregnancy can cause severe congenital abnormality in the baby. In England and Wales in 1986, there were 196 confirmed cases of rubella infection in pregnancy (DHSS, 1986[1]). Many of the pregnancies were terminated.

In any district, the District Health Authority (DHA) has responsibility for rubella immunization of schoolgirls. If parents choose to have their child immunized by the general practitioner and not the DHA, the practice does not always know that it is responsible. Moreover, as the DHA does not always inform the practice when it immunizes a schoolgirl, practice records may be incomplete.

Reason for the audit

Partners were aware that some of their female patients, certain of whom had not been schoolgirls in their district, were having their first test for rubella immunity as part of routine blood testing during their first pregnancy, which is too late.

Previous practice policy was to test all women for rubella immunity when they attended for contraceptive advice and to record rubella status on the patients' manual records. The partners and practice administrator thought that policy and implementation were inadequate, but did not know to what extent. In addition, the retrieval of information from manual records was sometimes difficult.

For 9 months, the partners had been transferring data onto a practice computer on an 'opportunistic' basis, i.e. as patients attended. From a starting point of zero records, they did not know what they had achieved.

Aims of audit

1 To determine the percentage of schoolgirls aged 13 years on the practice list who had been immunized against rubella, to compare the figure with national and local averages, and to agree upon measures that would improve uptake.
2 To determine the percentage of women aged 16–39 years who had not been sterilized or who had had a hysterectomy whose rubella status was recorded on the practice computer (practice policy).
3 To agree upon necessary steps to improve the testing and recording of rubella status.

Success was ascertained by comparing practice schoolgirl immunization figures with DHA and UK averages; rubella status figures were compared with the target of 100% recorded immunity for women aged 16–39 years at risk of pregnancy.

Methods

The practice administrator undertook a computer search to identify school-girls born in 1977, and identified who had had immunizations recorded. He then compared these data with the DHA records of rubella immunization of the same girls.

For the rubella status audit of women aged 16–39 years, the practice administrator undertook four computer searches for: the total number; rubella status; hysterectomy history; and sterilization history.

Who carried out the audit?

The audit was designed by the partner who took overall responsibility, but it was carried out by the practice administrator.

Results

Immunization of schoolgirls

The results showed that immunization levels for schoolgirls were below the national and district average (Table CS14.1). The disparity between

Table CS14.1   Immunization of girls aged 13 years (all born in 1977)

	No.	%
Total	26	
Number shown on practice computer as having been vaccinated	20	77
Number shown on DHA computer as having been vaccinated	21	81
DHA average		97*
UK average		86*

*Uptake in girls by 14th birthday.

DHA figures for uptake of immunization in the practice and in the district is surprising because the DHA is responsible for both. This difference may reflect the small number of girls being immunized in the practice or cast doubt on the high 97% uptake for the district. As the practice team achieves its other immunization targets, there is no reason to suspect unusually poor compliance in the practice population.

Although the denominators are slightly different for the practice and the DHA and UK (girls born in 1977 for the practice, girls who have reached their 14th birthday for DHA and UK figures), analysis of the data revealed that this difference did not affect the results.

Recording of rubella status ages 16–39 years.

The results of audit of rubella status reflect 9 months' work recording rubella status; after a further 6 weeks, the rate of recording increased from 34.5% in 9 months (3.8% per month) to 8.5% in 6 weeks (6.1% per month) (*see* Table CS14.2).

The data do not permit distinction between lack of testing and lack of recording. As the figures for hysterectomy had already been scrutinized as

Table CS14.2   Rubella status in women aged 16–39 years

	No.	%	No. at 6 weeks	%
Total	758		752	
Number recorded as having had hysterectomy	9		9	
Number recorded has having been sterilized	8		9	
Number of women aged 16–39 years who have no computer record of sterilization or hysterectomy	741		734	
Of this group, number whose rubella status is recorded	256	34.5	316	43

part of the cervical cytology screening programme, they were more likely to be complete than figures for sterilization and rubella status.

The results answer the question posed. The practice team was able to compare its results with local and national figures and identify opportunities for improvement.

Changes resulting from audit

At a practice meeting following the baseline audits of girls and women, the following changes were agreed.

1 In addition to DHA policy, the practice would attempt to ensure that every girl registered with the practice is immunized against rubella before her 14th birthday.
2 The practice administrator would regularly monitor immunization of 13-year-old girls, obtaining DHA information where necessary. It is also his responsibility to ensure that girls who have not been immunized are offered immunization and that partners follow up defaulters.
3 All women in the age-group 16–39 years should have recorded on the practice computer that they have had a hysterectomy, been sterilized or are rubella-immune. It is the responsiblity of the doctor or nurse who last saw the patient to ensure that the necessary recording or testing is carried out.
4 All women in the age-group 16–39 years who have not had a hysterectomy or been sterilized and whose rubella status is unknown should be offered testing on an opportunistic basis. If they decline testing, this should be clearly noted.

Was the audit repeated?

The audit will be repeated in 1 year, during which period continued progress is anticipated.

Comment

The overall aim of reducing the risk of a child being born with congenital rubella syndrome is worthwhile on both humane and economic grounds.

The ultimate outcome of the success of a rubella immunization programme would be to count the number of babies affected by congenital rubella syndrome and the number of terminations performed due to rubella infection during pregnancy. Although such an audit might be useful on a national or regional scale, it would be of little value to an individual practice in which there had been few cases per year for many years. Owing to the small denominator, measures of intermediate outcome were selected for which a standard could be set and progress measured.

The results enabled the partners and practice administrator to identify weaknesses (e.g. the transfer of information from the DHA and the follow-up of immunization defaulters) and to decide upon measures to achieve the agreed standards. The practice team could also assess the progress made in entering information into a relatively new computer system.

Although the results show that work needs to be done to implement the practice's own standards, procedures have been agreed upon and progress assessed.

Case Study 15

Subject of audit

THE audits of the care of patients with diabetes in a general practice were intended to improve glycaemic control and thereby reduce the risk of complications.

Background

Three audits were carried out in a practice of 4500 patients with 47 known patients with diabetes (1.1% of the practice population); 12 patients who regularly attend a consultant diabetic clinic were excluded.

With approximately two new cases diagnosed each year and a fairly stable population (total practice turnover of patients 5% per annum), the group of patients studied, i.e. the denominator, remained reasonably constant.

The first audit in 1986 led to the partners defining a protocol for the care of patients (Appendix 1) and agreeing that they would continue to see patients with diabetes during regular surgery sessions. The second audit in 1987 led to the institution of a regular practice diabetic clinic and a new protocol (Appendix 2). The third audit reviewed the diabetic control of patients attending the diabetic clinic.

Reasons for the audit

The first audit had shown that glycaemic control of practice patients with diabetes was unsatisfactory and that important observations (e.g. weight, smoking history, fundoscopy and foot examination) were either not being carried out or not being recorded. The second audit showed that the first protocol did not produce much improvement.

Aim of the audit

The aim was to see how closely the practice team complied with its protocol for the care of patients with diabetes, and to assess the effectiveness of the diabetic clinic.

The audit measured the percentage of patients for whom essential data was recorded at least annually, and compared three parameters (blood pressure, glycosylated haemoglobin and weight) against ideal levels.

Methods

Patients suffering from diabetes were identified from the practice disease index. To ensure that the list was complete, a computer search was also carried out to find all patients receiving prescriptions for insulin, oral hypoglycaemic agents and Diastix (urine glucose testing sticks). (Now that blood glucose monitoring equipment is available on prescription a search could also be made for BM-test strips, etc.)

One partner reviewed the records of every patient with diabetes for each of the three audits, to ensure consistency. A dedicated diabetic record card had been introduced into each patient's notes when the diabetic clinic was started, so these were easy to count.

Who carried out the audit?

The partner responsible for the organization and effectiveness of the care of patients with diabetes, and now responsible for the diabetic clinic, was responsible for the audit. (Now that systems are established for recording data and less searching of records is necessary, it should be possible to delegate further audits to practice staff.)

Results

The results of recording of data for the three audits are given in Table CS15.1. The relevant audit dates are 1986 (before protocol agreed), 1987 (before clinic established), and 1989 (clinic running).

Intermediate outcome measurements of clinical management between 1987 and 1989 (i.e. before and after the commencement of the diabetic clinic) are shown in Table CS15.2.

The results show that the first set of criteria and standards did not result in much improvement in the process of care, as measured by the recorded data; there were fewer recordings of examination of patients' feet for evidence of complications.

Table CS15.1   Data from all three audits

	Percentage recorded		
	1986	1987	1989
1 Evidence of diagnosis	91	100	100
2 Ideal weight	12	12	100
3 Diet	21	21	100
4 Smoking history	14	14	100
5 Treatment	97	97	100
6 Visual acuity	2	20	96
7 Appearance of optic fundi	12	24	96
8 Foot examination	25	16	96
9 Urinalysis	51	60	96
10 Random blood glucose*	57	56	0
11 Glycosylated Hb	40	68	96
12 Weight	34	56	96
13 Blood pressure	76	84	96

*Random blood glucose deleted from the statement of practice policy as glycosylated Hb gives more useful information.

Table CS15.2 Intermediate outcome measures of clinical management between 1987 and 1989

	Worse	No change	Improvement
Glycosylated Hb	57%	22%	21%
Weight	31%	19%	50%
Blood pressure	41%	39%	20%

However, the third audit revealed a considerable improvement in recording once the diabetic clinic had been established, a revised protocol agreed upon and care shared with a nurse, dietitian and chiropodist. Despite this apparent improvement in process, changes in intermediate outcome measures (glycosylated haemoglobin, weight and blood pressure) were disappointing.

Changes resulting from audit

Following the third and most recent audit, the doctors, nurse, dietitian and chiropodist reviewed the data and decided to take a more aggressive approach towards dietary advice, hypoglycaemic therapy and blood pressure control. The success (or otherwise) of this policy will be revealed by the next audit.

Comment

This is an example of an audit of chronic disease management using data from the clinical record (*see* Chapter 7). The same format could be used to audit other chronic conditions, such as asthma and hypertension.

In this case, outcome could have been audited by measuring the prevalence and severity of complications (which will be done), but numbers are small and the results will be subject to wide statistical error. For example, visual acuity could be compared yearly or the number of digits possessed by each patients could be counted and compared with the number possessed last year. Frequency of hospitalization or hypoglycaemia could also be measured.

However, it is easy to record data and do nothing about it. The blood pressure of the entire practice population may be recorded but unless those patients with abnormal levels are investigated and treated their risk of complications will not be reduced. Similarly, taking blood to test for glycosylated haemoglobin and recording the result does not reduce a diabetic patient's chance of becoming blind. These particular audits of diabetes are an example of a pleasing process audit hiding unsatisfactory intermediate outcome results (*see* Chapter 3).

Appendix CS15.1: Diabetic protocol (written after first audit)

Protocol for recording

The following data should be recorded in the notes of all patients of diabetes.

Recorded once

- Evidence of diagnosis
- Ideal weight
- Diet (CHO)
- Smoking history

Recorded within the last year

- Description of treatment
- Blood sugar
- Glycosylated haemoglobin
- Visual acuity
- Peripheral pulses
- Evidence of neuropathy
- Date and severity of last hypoglycaemic attack (particularly drivers)

Recorded each visit (for whatever reason)

- Weight
- Blood pressure
- Urinalysis

Appendix CS15.2: Diabetic protocol (written after second audit)

Protocol for diabetic clinic

1 Timing
Clinic held third Tuesday every month 3.00–6.00 pm.
Annual 30-minute appointment.

2 Patients
All patients with diabetes not regularly seen at a hospital diabetic clinic.

3 Nurse
Record on green card:

- Date
- Height
- Weight
- Ideal weight (see obesity protocol for ideal weights)
- Corrected visual acuity, each eye
- Urine test for glucose, protein, blood, ketones

Arrange MSU if urine shows protein or blood
Complete green biochemistry card ticking glycosylated haemoglobin and creatinine.

Dilate pupils
Instil 1 drop 0.5% tropicaimide into each eye unless there is a dense cataract, glaucoma, history of eye surgery, pain or redness.
Consult doctor if unsure.

4 Doctor
Record on green card:

Blood pressure (see centile chart)
Condition of leg and foot pulses
Knee, ankle and plantar reflexes
Vibration and light touch senses knees, ankles and feet
Condition of fundi, particularly signs of retinopathy
Presence and severity of cataracts
Refer to eye clinic if retinopathy seen or cataract surgery necessary
Take blood for glycosylated haemoglobin and creatinine
Request random serum cholesterol if (a) not measured within past 5 years or (b) previous level > 6.5 mmol/l
Reinforce general health advice (see Well Person Protocols *re* smoking, alcohol, etc.)

Write to or phone each patient when blood results are available
Note history of hypoglycaemic attacks

5 Dietitian and chiropodist
All patients should see dietitian and chiropodist each year

6 Diagnosis
Random blood glucose > 11.0 mmol/l

7 Management
Aim for random blood glucose < 10.0 mmol/l (preferably 8.0 mmol/l)
and gly Hb < 9.0% mmol/l

Type I diabetes

- Refer newly diagnosed patients to consultant physician diabetic clinic for
  initial treatment
- Adjust insulin and diet in cooperation with dietitian
- Refer back to consultant physician diabetic clinic if control difficult or
  poor
- Encourage regular body mass monitoring at home

Type II diabetes (without ketonuria)

- Prescribe diet alone in first instance if weight 15% above ideal
- Repeat gly Hb and urinalysis in 1 month
- If uncontrolled continue dietary advice and prescribe:
  metformin 500 mg b.d. (if patient obese and serum creatinin normal);
  or gliclazide (Diamicron R 80 mg), initially 40–80 mg daily (maximum
  320 mg, 4 tablets daily)
- Do not change an existing patient from glibenclamide (maximum 15 mg,
  3 tablets daily) to gliclazide unless he/she has hypoglycaemic symptoms
- Consider referral to consultant physician diabetic clinic if glycosylated
  haemoglobin remains > 9.0%

References

Chapter 3

1 Royal College of General Practitioners (1985) *Quality in general practice* Policy Statement 2. RCGP, London.
2 Secretaries of State for Health, England, Wales, Northern Ireland and Scotland (1989) *Working for patients* (Cmd 555). HMSO, London.
3 Shaw C and Costain D W (1989) Guidelines for medical audit: seven principles. *Brit Med J.*, **299**, 498–9.
4 Hughes J and Humphrey C (1990) *Medical audit in general practice: a practical guide to the literature.* King Edward's Hospital Fund for London, London.
5 Donabedian A (1966) Evaluating the quality of medical care. *Millbank Memorial Fund Quarterly.* **44**, 166–204.
6 Buck C, Fry J and Irvine D H (1974) A framework for good primary care: the measurement and achievement of quality. *J R Coll Gen Pract.* **24**, 599–604.

Chapter 4

1 Thornham R (1990) Audit and performance review. *Practice Update.* **44**, 1033–8.
2 Ashton J *et al.*, (1976) An audit of deaths in general practice. *Update.* **12**, 1019–22.
3 Irvine D H *et al.*, (1986) Educational development and evaluation research in the Northern region. In: Pendleton D, Schofield T, Marinker M (Eds) *In pursuit of quality.* RCGP, London.
4 Grol R *et al.*, (1988) Peer review in general practice: methods, standards, protocols. University Department of General Practice, Niemegen.
5 (1957) *Report on Public Health and Medical Subjects* No. 97. HMSO, London.
6 (1960) *Report on Public Health and Medical Subjects* No. 103. HMSO, London.
7 Buck C *et al.*, (1987) *Confidential enquiry into perioperative deaths.* Nuffield Provincial Hospital Trust, London.
8 Joint Commitee on Postgraduate Training for General Practice (1987) *Assessment of vocational training for general practice.* Final report of JCPTGP Working Party, available on request.

Chapter 5

1 Baker R and Presley P (1990) *The practice audit plan: a handbook of medical audit.* RCGP Severn Faculty, Bristol.
2 Russell D and Russell I (1990) Statistical issues in medical audit, In: Marinker M (Ed) *Medical audit in general practice.* BMJ for MSD Foundation, London.

Chapter 6

1 North of England Study of Standards and Performance in General Practice (1990) *Setting clinical standards within small groups* (Vol. I) Final Report No. 40. Health Care Research Unit, Newcastle upon Tyne.
2 Schoenbaum S C and Gottlieb L K (1990) Algorithms based on improvement of clinical quality. *Brit Med J*. **301**, 1374–6.
3 British Medical Journal (1989) *Clinical algorithms: gynaecology*. BMJ, London.
4 Royal College of General Practitioners Clinical Folders: Diabetes (2nd edn 1988); Asthma (1987); Coronary heart disease (1988); Parkinsons disease (1987); Epilepsy (1987); Rheumatoid arthritis (1989); Terminal care (1990); Depression (1989). RCGP, London.

Chapter 7

1 Crombie D and Fleming D (1988) *Practice activity analysis*. Occasional Paper 41. RCGP, London.
2 Abrahamson J H (1987) *Survey methods in community medicine*. Churchill Livingstone, London.
3 Royal College of General Practitioners (1985) *What sort of doctor?* Report from general practice No. 23. RCGP, London.

Chapter 8

1 Royal College of General Practitioners (1990) *Who killed Susan Thompson?* Video and coursebook. MSD Foundation for RCGP, London.
2 (1957) *Report on Public Health and Medical Subjects* No. 97. HMSO, London.
3 (1960) *Report on Public Health and Medical Subjects* No. 103. HMSO, London.
4 Buck C *et al.*, (1987) *Confidential enquiry into perioperative deaths*. Nuffield Provincial Hospital Trust, London.
5 Personal communication, Northumberland DHA.
6 Kessner D M *et al.*, (1973) Assessing health quality: the case for tracers. *N Engl J Med*. **288**, 189–94.
7 Royal College of General Practitioners (1985) *What sort of doctor?* Report from general practice No. 23. RCGP, London.
8 Royal College of General Practitioners (1990) *Fellowship by assessment*, Occasional paper 50. RCGP, London.

Chapter 9

1 Dean A D *et al.*, (1990) EpiInfo, Version 5: a word processing data base, and statistics programme for epidemiology on microcomputers. Center for Disease Control, Atlanta.

Chapter 10

1 Gregsen B A *et al.*, (1991) *Interprofessional collaboration between health care organizations.* Occasional paper 52. RCGP, London.
2 Huntington J (1991) Personal communication.
3 Irvine D (1990) *Managing for quality in general practice.* King Edward's Hospital Fund for London, London.
4 Adelaide Medical Centre Primary Health Care Team (1991) A primary health care team manifesto. *Brit J Gen Pract.* **41**, 31–5.
5 Irvine, S (1987) Delegation: the manager's nightmare. *Horizons.* **10**, 530–8.
6 Plant R (1987) *Managing change and making it stick.* Collins, London.

Chapter 11

1 General Medical Council (1991) *Professional conduct and discipline: fitness to practice.* GMC, London.
2 United Kingdom Council for Nursing, Midwifery and Health Visiting (1984) *Code of Professional Conduct for the Nurse, Midwife and Health Visitor.* UKCC, London.
3 General Medical Council (1987) *Annual Report for 1986.* GMC, London.
4 Department of Health (1990) *Medical audit in the family practitioner services.* Health Circular (FP)(90)8. HMSO, London.
5 Department of Health (1991) *Medical audit in the hospital and community services.* Health Circular (91)(2). HMSO, London.

Chapter 12

1 Hadfield, S J (1953) A field survey of general practice. *Brit Med J.* **2**, 683–706.
2 Taylor, S (1954) *Good general practice.* Oxford University Press for Nuffield Provincial Hospital Trust, London.
3 Collings J S (1950) General practice in England today. *The Lancet.* **1**, 555–85.
4 Irvine D H and Jeffreys M (1971) BMA Planning Unit survey of general practice. *Brit Med J.* **4**, 535–43.
5 Peterson O L *et al.*, (1956) An analytical study of North Carolina general practice 1953–54. *Journal of Medical Education.* **31**, 12(2).
6 Clute L F (1963) *The general practitioner.* University of Toronto Press, London.
7 Jungfer C C and Last J M (1964) Clinical performance in Australian general practice. *Medicine.* **2**, 71–83.
8 Barley S L and Mathers N (1980) An audit of the care of post-gastrectomy patients. *J R Coll Gen Prac.* **30**, 365–70.
9 Colmer L J and Gray D J P (1983) An audit of the care of asthma in general practice. *The Practitioner.* **227**, 271–9.
10 Hart J T H (1975) The management of high blood pressure in general practice. *J R Coll Gen Pract.* **25**, 160–92.
11 Marsh G N (1977) Obstetric audit in general practice. *Brit Med J.* **2**, 1004–6.

12 Hughes J and Humphreys C (1990) *Medical audit in general practice: a practical guide to the literature*. King Edward's Hospital Fund for London, London.
13 Department of Health (1990) *Medical audit in the family practitioner services*. Health Circular (FP)(90)8. HMSO, London.

Case Study 8

1 Royal College of General Practitioners (1985) *Quality in general practice*. Policy statement 2. RCGP, London.
2 Fraser R C (1987) *Clinical method: a general practice approach*. Butterworth, London.
3 Drury M (1990) (Ed) *The new practice manager*. Radcliffe Medical Press, Oxford.

Case Study 9

1 Petrie J C *et al.*, (1986) British Hypertension Society: recommendations on blood pressure measurement. *Brit Med J*. **293**, 611–15.
2 Swales, J D *et al.*, (1989) British Hypertension Society Working Party: treating mild hypertension. *Brit Med J*. **298**, 694–8.
3 Hart J T (1970) Semicontinuous screening of a whole community for hypertension. *The Lancet*. **2**, 223–6.
4 Hart J T (1987) *Hypertension* (2nd edn). Churchill Livingstone, London.
5 Jewell D and Hope J (1988) Evaluation of a nurse run hypertension clinic in general practice. *The Practitioner*. 484–7.
6 Medical Research Council Working Party (1985) MRC trial of treating mild hypertension: principal results. *Brit Med J*. **291**, 97.
7 De Souza M F, Swan A V, Shannon D J (1976) A long term controlled trial of screening for hypertension in general practice. *The Lancet*. **1**, 1228–31.

Case Study 13

1 Wilkin D and Smith A A (1987) A variation in general practitioners' referral rates to consultants. *J R Coll Gen Pract*. **37**, 350–3.

Case Study 14

1 Department of Health and Social Security (1986) *On the state of public health: annual report of chief medical officer of DHSS*. HMSO, London.

Index